Recreation, Leisure and Chronic Illness: Therapeutic Rehabilitation as Intervention in Health Care

Recreation, Leisure and Chronic Illness: Therapeutic Rehabilitation as Intervention in Health Care

Miriam P. Lahey, Robin Kunstler, Arnold H. Grossman,
Frances Daly, Stuart Waldman, Fred Schwartz
Editors

The Haworth Press, Inc.
New York • London • Norwood (Australia)

Recreation, Leisure and Chronic Illness: Therapeutic Rehabilitation as Intervention in Health Care has also been published as *Loss, Grief & Care* , Volume 6, Number 4 1993.

The Haworth Press, Inc., 10 Alice Street, Binghamton, NY 13904-1580 USA

Library of Congress Cataloging-in-Publication Data

Recreation, leisure and chronic illness: therapeutic rehabilitation as intervention in health care/Miriam P. Lahey . . . [et al.], editors.
    p. cm.
    "Has also been published as Loss, grief & care, v. 6, no. 4, 1993"-T.p. verso.
    Includes bibliographical references.
    ISBN 1-56024-418-6 (acid-free)
    1. Recreational therapy. I. Lahey, Miriam P.
RM736.7.R43 1992
615.8'5153–dc20

                                                   93-16983
                                                     CIP

Recreation, Leisure and Chronic Illness: Therapeutic Rehabilitation as Intervention in Health Care

CONTENTS

Preface xi

Acknowledgments xix

Trends That Affect Quality of Life: Recreation as a Tool for Enhancement 1
Frances Wallach

Environment 2
Economics 3
Users 4
Political Impact 5
Professional Image 5

Work, Health, and Recreation: Aspects of the Total Person 7
Michael K. Bartalos

Assumptions 8
Life Plan of the Individual 8
Adaptation to the Environment 9
Mental Attitude as an Adaptive Tool 9
Work and Leisure as Adaptive Activities 10
Stress as an Adaptive Mechanism 11
Components of Adaptation 11
Benefits of Recreational Activities 12

Choice of Recreational Activities 13
Conclusion 14

**Balancing Changing Health Care Needs
with the Shortage of Quality Health Care
Professionals: Implications for Therapeutic Recreation** **15**
Peg Connolly

The Profession of Therapeutic Recreation 17
Shortage of Qualified Health Care Professionals 18
Conclusion 21

**Clinical Effectiveness of Intensive Therapeutic
Recreation: A Multiple Case Study
of Private Practice Intervention** **23**
Robin Kunstler
Steven Sokoloff

**Quality of Living Until Death: A Fusion of Death
Awareness into Therapeutic Recreation-Leisure
Education** **31**
Carol Stensrud

The "Why" of Death Awareness 33
Settings and Populations Addressed 33
Values of Death Awareness 34
A Comparison of Death Awareness and Leisure Education 35
The Leisure Link 36
Therapeutic Recreation Professionals Address Death 36
Lifeline Activity 37

**Psychosocial Issues Confronting Health Care
Professionals Working with People with AIDS** **39**
Arnold H. Grossman

Some Assumptions 39
Blaming the Victim 40
Role of the Therapeutic Recreation Specialist 42

Psychosocial Issues   43
Conclusion   48

Occupational Therapy Intervention in Recreational Activities in Acute Care Settings   **51**
Ann Burkhardt

Acute Care vs. Chronic Care Models of Service to the Elderly: Implications for Therapeutic Recreation   **55**
Miriam P. Lahey

Therapeutic Recreation: Competing Models of the Profession   56
The Chronic Care Needs of the Elderly   57
Acute Care vs. Chronic Care in the United States   59
The Advent of DRGs   61
DRGs: The Impact on Therapeutic Recreation   62

Surviving a Fate Worse than Death: The Plight of the Homebound Elderly   **67**
Stuart Waldman

Therapeutic Group Activities with Alzheimer's Patients   **73**
Sidney R. Saul

Meaningful Life Activities for Elderly Residents of Residential Health Care Facilities   **79**
Shura Saul

From Custodial Care to Quality Care: Implications for the Therapeutic Recreation Professional   **87**
Fred S. Greenblatt

What Is Quality Care?   89
Quality Assurance   90
The State Survey Process: Historical Perspectives   91
Implications for Therapeutic Recreation   96

**The Therapeutic Value of Art for Persons
with Alzheimer's Disease and Related Disorders**   **99**
Jane E. Harlan

**The Effectiveness of Cueing on Anagram Solving
by Cognitively Impaired Nursing Home Elderly**   **107**
Kestal T. Phillips

Hypotheses   107
Definition of Terms   108
Review of the Literature   108
Methods   110
Results and Interpretation of Findings   112
Limitations   115

Recreation in the Nursing Home   **117**
Elaine Streitfeld

Playing for Keeps   **127**
Michael Spiegel

 ALL HAWORTH BOOKS & JOURNALS
ARE PRINTED ON CERTIFIED
ACID-FREE PAPER

ABOUT THE EDITORS

Miriam P. Lahey, PhD, is Coordinator, Recreation Program, Department of Physical Education, Recreation and Dance, Division of Professional Studies, Lehman College of CUNY, Bronx, New York.

Robin Kunstler, REd, is Coordinator, Recreation Department, Lehman College of CUNY, Bronx, New York.

Arnold H. Grossman, PhD, CSW, CLP, is Chairman and Professor, Recreation and Leisure Studies, School of Education, Health, Nursing and Arts Professions, New York University, New York, New York.

Frances Daly, MS, is Past President, Metropolitan New York Parks and Recreation Association, New York, New York, and is Professor, Recreation Program, Department of Physical Education, Recreation and Dance, Division of Professional Studies, Lehman College of CUNY, Bronx, New York.

Stuart Waldman, MS, is Director of Activities, Menorah Home and Hospital, Brooklyn, New York.

Fred Schwartz, CSW, is a Caseworker for Catholic Guardian Society, Missionaries of Charity, and was formerly Recreation Therapist, Memorial Sloan-Kettering Cancer Center (Pediatric Oncology), New York, New York.

Preface

This volume represents a collaboration between the Foundation of Thanatology at Columbia University and the Recreation Department at Lehman College of the City University of New York. The intent of this collaboration was to bridge the gap between the fields of leisure and thanatology. Obviously, this meant a concern with the intersecting issues of leisure and dying, issues that are not often explored either by leisure professionals or those concerned with death and dying.

We sought a collaboration, however, that would go beyond a focus on the meaning of leisure in the midst of life-threatening illness. The focus of the Foundation of Thanatology was our guide here. The Foundation is concerned not only with conditions that threaten the quantity of life but also those that threaten its quality. Life-threatening conditions are understood to include not only illnesses, but social, psychological, economic, and environmental conditions as well. The Foundation therefore encourages exploration of all avenues of intervention that support the quality as well as the quantity of life. In linking leisure and thanatology, it is crucial, then, to reflect on the role of recreation in the rehabilitation of those whose lives are threatened with a wide range of diminishments.

Although philosophies of leisure abound, all of them agree that freedom is central to true leisure, as is enjoyment, self-determination, and some experience of transcendence, of breaking through the routines and set patterns of daily existence. The studies in this collection all explore this general definition, but do so within a wide variety of settings and in the face of multiple threats to both the quantity and quality of life.

Frances Wallach describes leisure as a mode of life enhancement. When illness, disability, stress, or poverty threaten the quantity or quality of a person's life, leisure often takes on great meaning. Because it is central to personal identity, the continuation of leisure pursuits can sustain personal history and compensate when other life roles are disrupted. Moreover, by interjecting the non-seriousness of play, leisure can provide a saving balance in the midst of serious illness or disability. This is particularly important in the clinical milieu. Finally, leisure skills signal mastery and accomplishment, which can contribute to rebuilding confidence eroded by sickness or stress. Indeed, as Michael K. Bartalos points out, leisure is closely intertwined with health and work in sustaining the quality of life. It is therefore a positive counterforce to the diminishments that erode health and work.

Under normal conditions, of course, people are capable of managing their own leisure, as they manage other areas of life. In fact, leisure is a value precisely because it allows individuals to pursue personally chosen, self-managed activity. When overcome by limiting conditions, however, individuals may need help in realizing this fundamental value. Peg Connolly offers insight on how recreation professionals, specially trained to facilitate the leisure experiences of their clients, can respond to such threatening situations. Here, the nature of therapeutic recreation as a helping profession is clearly exhibited.

The commitment to "help" is, of course, rooted in the history of the recreation movement, a history that can be traced back to the social reform movements of the late nineteenth century and a special concern for the poor. The plight of those condemned to overcrowded urban centers and dehumanizing industrial working conditions prompted the demand for leisure services that would provide opportunities for relaxation and personal growth in both community and institutional settings. Out of that beginning, distinctly separate recreation services arose–community or municipal recreation, which focused on leisure as a basic human right, and therapeutic recreation, which split into two areas, one focusing on the therapeutic benefits of leisure experience, with emphasis on leisure experience, the other on recreation as an intervention tool, with emphasis on therapeutic outcome.

In 1961 the American Medical Association officially designated recreation services as an allied health field. The profession was thus formally recognized as part of the health care system, and since then it has sought to demonstrate its clinical effectiveness in terms of the medical model. Even community or municipal recreation services define their role largely in terms of promoting a healthy life-style. This dependency on the medical model has, however, contributed to a sense of professional diffidence in the field of recreation because its role is so clearly ancillary to the medical and nursing professions.

Furthermore, the medical model is an *acute-care* model which has been persistently unresponsive to those who suffer from chronic illness, mental and emotional disabilities, and the health care risks that are rooted in social conditions. As Miriam Lahey points out, this model is not responsive to major groups of clients served by the leisure professions: the elderly, the children of the poor, at-risk youth, the homeless, the medically uninsured, and other groups within the population who are left at the margins of health care policy.

The funding of the health care system is an additional problem. Third-party reimbursement for health care services rarely recognizes the part played by recreation in promoting and restoring health; almost never does it cover the costs of such services when rendered outside the clinical setting. This is because funding agencies generally perceive leisure as a luxury that should be paid for privately, rather than as a basic human necessity to be included under the entitlements of the health care system. Yet the psychosocial benefits from recreation services have been clearly documented. Not only does recreation provide diversion from pain and stress, but the leisure experience can play a major part in rehabilitation through building confidence and self-esteem, as Robin Kunstler and Steven Sokoloff illustrate.

The limits of the acute-care model argue for a more holistic vision of health care, one focused on total well-being, rather than simply the absence of disease. In such a model, all that enhances growth, all that promotes life, would have place. A humanistic-holistic perspective would recognize the need of persons to make choices, to exercise freedom, to grow and develop as individuals. In such a perspective, leisure education would be an important element in building the human person and human society. Such an approach treats the whole person rather than disease, and measures its gains in terms of peoples' ability to take responsibility for their own needs.

A humanistic-holistic model of health care addresses clients' needs in a variety of settings, rather than limiting service to the acute-care hospital. Stuart Waldman indicates how, in some alternate settings, the opportunity for leisure is limited by illness, poverty, stress, or other oppressive conditions. In these settings, as Michael Spiegel indicates, improvement in leisure life-style can serve as a crucial first step in rehabilitation.

While the medical model limits its perception of service setting to hospitals, a broader perspective would recognize that threats to quality and quantity of life frequently are found in the community setting. Persons struggling with life-threatening conditions are in parks and playgrounds, in shopping malls and in health clubs. Arnold Grossman, for example, deals with the part played by recreation in the lives of persons with AIDS, a disease which often brings people into hospitals, but which also finds them trying to cope with life in their community. Because of the fears and faulty information about AIDS, there is often difficulty in integrating AIDS patients into community groups for recreation. Part of the leisure professional's role is to educate groups about the disease so that patients can remain part of the community leisure experience.

The elderly constitute another group with special health needs. Leisure services are very important for the quality of life of the young-old who are newly retired, as well as for the very old, who make up the fastest-growing segment of the population. Recreation programs in senior centers provide much-needed opportunity to maintain social skills, prevent depression, and develop a sense of achievement and control. Increasingly, the thrust of service provision for the elderly is directed to home care and day care, which call for a wide spectrum of services and caregivers, including recreation professionals. In such community-based programs, leisure services form an important part of a care model in which the emphasis is on preserving existing coping patterns and preventing decline of functioning.

For those elderly who can no longer be sustained at home, nursing home placement is sometimes the only practical alternative. This is especially so since Medicare now exerts tremendous pressure for early hospital discharge of the elderly. For those elderly who are discharged "quicker and sicker" from hospitals, nursing homes are often the only viable option. But planning recreation programs for these very sick–and institutionalized–older people presents many challenges. The freedom and choice central to leisure experience is drastically limited for many of these elderly, and the frequency of cognitive impairment creates additional demands for creative program development.

Jane Harlan and Elaine Streitfeld report on programs that have been successful with the elderly suffering from Alzheimer's disease and related disorders. Frequently, these persons are perceived as being beyond rehabilitation, yet, in spite of their cognitive losses they have a wealth of affective resources at their disposal–resources that can be tapped in a good recreation program. Carefully structured programs for these clients not only help to preserve their functioning, but also provide respite for family caregivers. While the patients' conditions cannot be reversed, their fears and sense of isolation can be alleviated, and their memory function strengthened through appropriate expressive activities and regular group participation.

Patients in psychiatric hospitals also need help with cognitive functioning, as well as affective and social functioning. Many of these patients have a high rate of recidivism, and, along with their families and caregivers, they often begin to lose hope for change in their lives. As Michael Spiegel illustrates, recreation is often able to break this cycle of failure when other interventions have failed. This may be because recreation is seen by the patients as less threatening and less judgmental, or perhaps it is because they can more readily achieve success in their leisure than in their work or family roles. Leisure counseling plays an important part in discharge planning for psychiatric patients, since even those who are successful in their employment find managing their evenings and weekends very difficult.

For those suffering from terminal illnesses in hospital or hospice settings, the meaning of leisure is often misunderstood. In the prevailing acute-care model, death is serious business; it leaves little room for play or fun or enjoyment. Yet those who are dying can find meaning in the leisure values which have nourished them throughout their life. Indeed, the transcendent function of leisure can be very important for those searching for life's ultimate meaning in the face of death. Since the threat of death poses the greatest possible challenge to one's sense of identity, those leisure pursuits which have contributed powerfully to self-identification will be particularly meaningful at this time. This theme is explored by Carol Stensrud, who focuses on the relationship between leisure education and death education.

Not only do leisure services include a number of different client groups, they also involve a variety of activities. Various authors provide evidence of the power of music, dance, art and creative writing activities to draw people out of depression, to facilitate appropriate social interaction, to stimulate memory, to release feelings, to focus attention.

Music, whether enjoyed alone or in large groups, whether performed or listened to, has indeed the power to charm. Even those with very limited language capacity can respond to music. In short, music features prominently in recreation groups for every age group and setting.

Dance programs too, have great appeal and are especially important in developing the whole person. Dance as expressive movement to music can bring a sense of freedom to the performer and the viewer. Even those whose physical condition precludes their taking part in the dance can vicariously share the freedom of motion when watching dance performances.

For those whose cognitive, and especially language skills are impaired, working with color, line and form in art activities can provide an enjoyable medium for release of impacted feelings. Here, success is measured not so much by the skill of the client as by the sense of achievement and pleasure. Again, the enjoyment can come from a wide range of art activities, from active creation to viewing slides or pictures of others' work. It can be a solitary, silent experience, or can be shared in making a group project. Through art, one learns to risk, to show oneself, to experiment. It is an adventure which can bring great gains.

Creative writing, too, is a form of leisure experience which can have the added benefit of stimulating memory and helping to focus attention. Writing can help with cognitive functioning as well as expressing feeling. Writing can be very private, as in journals, or it can be shared through publication.

Some of the articles in this volume deal with policy issues, others describe specific programs; some are theoretical, others very practical. All of them show the healing power of leisure, healing greatly needed by those suffering from life-threatening conditions, whether medical, social, economic, or environmental.

Miriam P. Lahey

Acknowledgments

The publication of this book was supported in part by a grant from the Lucius N. Littauer Foundation.

The editors wish to acknowledge the support and encouragement of the Foundation of Thanatology in the preparation of this volume. All royalties from the sale of this book are assigned to the Foundation of Thanatology, a tax-exempt, not-for-profit, scientific and educational foundation.

Thanatology, a new subspecialty of medicine, is involved in applying the knowledge derived from scientific and humanistic inquiries to increase our understanding of the psychological aspects of dying; reactions to loss, death, and grief; and recovery from bereavement.

The Foundation of Thanatology is dedicated to advancing the cause of enlightened health care for terminally ill patients and their families. The Foundation's orientation is a positive one, based on fostering more mature acceptance and understanding of death and the problems of grief and advocating more effective and humane management and treatment of dying patients and their bereaved family members.

Trends That Affect Quality of Life:
Recreation as a Tool for Enhancement

Frances Wallach

Family structure is changing. Less than 11 percent of women are currently stereotypical housewives, and this is an aging population. One in three full-time homemakers is a woman aged 65 or older; more than half are over 55. The number of homemakers will shrink as older women are replaced by younger women who work. Nearly half of the working women regard their work as a career. Moreover, young housewives today feel they have a right to pursue activities outside the home. This will be a new focus for leisure services.

Working women are doing less in the home, and the share of housework done by the husband rises dramatically when the wife works full-time. This will mean less, or more concentrated, leisure participation by men.

There will be a continued rise in the number of single-parent families, broken families and unmarried households. A continued rapid growth of child care programs will still lag behind the need for child care, both for preschool children and for latch-key children.

The largest population growth will be in the over-sixty group, and this aging population will have more time to spend and more retirement income than ever before. On the other hand, health care costs will continue to rise, eating up a larger segment of this group's income.

There will be a rising birth rate, not because of an increase in fertility rates, but because the baby-boom generation is having children. The growing population is having children, but not at a rate

Frances Wallach, EdD, is Consultant and President, Total Recreation Management Inc., and Adjunct Assistant Professor, New York University, New York, NY.

1

proportionate to past years. In 1970 there were four million more children of school age (ages 5-17) than adults aged 25 to 44. Today there are 33 million more 25 to 44 year olds than children of school age.

There will be an increase in the number of single men who continue to live alone or with lovers. By 1995, fully 46 percent of all households are expected to be headed by a man or woman without a spouse. However, male household heads are primarily under 45 years of age, and half of those were never married. Nearly half the single woman household heads are over 65 and widowed. The two-earner family appears to be an accepted fact of life. It is unlikely to change.

There will be an increase in the AIDS population; in the mentally ill homeless; in the correctional institution population. There appears to be an increasing awareness (although perhaps not an actual increase) of child abuse, spouse abuse, and elder abuse. If no controls are found, there will be a significant rise in substance abuse, with dependencies becoming more severe as drugs become more potent and cheaper to obtain.

As family structures disintegrate, the number of identified at-risk youth will increase. It is also expected that racial tensions will continue to increase, unless effective interventions are found, over the next decade.

Americans will work harder and longer in the coming decade, with a prediction by some forecasting experts that we could be looking at 50-55 hour workweeks. "At home" leisure or "cocooning" is predicted to continue. Television viewing has stabilized, but, since 1980, there has been a 40 percent rise in in-ground swimming pools; home-delivery sales of food are growing twice as fast as takeout or "drive through"; pet ownership is at an all-time high; and there has been a 47 percent rise in retail sales of lawn and garden supplies since 1983.

ENVIRONMENT

Population will continue to increase in total numbers. Food sources, and the labor to maintain those sources, will decrease.

Water, ocean, and air pollution will affect the world. The "greenhouse effect" has already caused great concern, as has the effect of "acid rain." Toxic pollutants in the air from incineration and industry continue to increase, starting to infiltrate the food chain.

The protection of public lands, wilderness systems, and natural wildlife areas will be a major concern, both nationally and at the state level. Greater use of natural areas by the public will require attention.

If the federal government continues to decrease its influence at the state level, the responsibility of the state will increase to preserve and maintain the environment. If state responsibility decreases, not-for-profit organizations will be given greater responsibility.

ECONOMICS

Tourism has become a growing industry and a major economic influence, both nationally and locally. The revenues from the travel industry now represent a major source of income–in fact, in some areas, the primary source of income. Travel will continue to increase, as will all the leisure service components connected to tourism.

One of the largest components of the country's gross national product is the production of articles used in recreation, ranging from sports equipment to recreation vehicles, to athletic clothing, VCRs, compact discs, walkman radios. While the economy has an impact on governmental budgets for recreation, it has little effect on the individual's spending for recreation. Recreation, on the other hand, has a tremendous impact on the national economy. Today we spend more money on recreation products than on national defense, and this trend is expected to continue.

A new trend is gaining ground in the economy of leisure services–contractual services, or privatization. The operation of public facilities by private agents will grow because of greater effectiveness, leading to increased revenues, and tax-base support of private operators.

The trend toward fee-charging for leisure services will increase.

An affluent population will be more willing to pay for quality services. Theme parks and Disney Worlds came about because the public showed a willingness to pay for their recreation experiences. This trend will continue, as will the public interest in activities that require high-cost support (such as boating, skiing) and high-cost equipment (rock-climbing, ballooning).

The rift between the affluent and the poor will continue to grow. Leisure services to the poor will continue to be a major responsibility of the public agencies. The availability of leisure services will increase in importance as a tool in marketing the desirability of living in a community, joining a specific workplace, visiting a tourist attraction.

The issues of safety and liability should decrease over the next decade. The increased attention given to risk reduction by agencies, the improved products, and the training of staffs, will show results in the reduction of liability situations in recreation facilities. However, because of attitudes of the legal community and their aggressive directions, the risk of being sued might not necessarily be decreased.

It should be noted that while in 1962 there were 85,000 civil law suits filed, in 1982 there were 230,000. Today, one out of every 16 people in the nation files a lawsuit.

The weakening dollar will impact on and reduce foreign travel, but should encourage foreign tourism in the United States.

USERS

Fitness will continue to grow as a concern of the American public. The deepest emphasis on fitness will be for the 0-12 year-olds and the 45 and over age group.

The more affluent population will continue to withdraw from public agency recreation, to individual or private participation. The poorer populations will continue to depend upon the public agency for recreation. This population will continue to make heavy use of local facilities, because of lack of income to travel longer distances for recreation.

Organized sports will continue to be the most successful output of public agencies. Individual activities will help develop the strength of private facilities. Greater attention will be paid to the needs of the disabled, because the power base of this group is growing. It is expected that, as an organized group, the disabled will be more successful in obtaining their required leisure services.

Because of population changes, more emphasis will have to be given to leisure services for preschool and latch-key children, the elderly, at-risk youth, the AIDS population, and the homeless.

Recreation for the homebound will not be successfully provided by public agencies, who have found great difficulty in identifying this population. The focus in this area will probably be from the voluntary, specialized agencies who currently serve the various needs of the homebound.

POLITICAL IMPACT

The role of the federal government in public recreation concerns will decrease at the local and state levels. The federal government will concern itself primarily with the conservation of federal lands, and such global problems as pollution.

State recreation agencies, in addition to administering state lands, will take on a more directly supportive role with local leisure service providers, using special funding such as bond issues. This support will include both financial and technical assistance.

Rural recreation agencies will face greater difficulties in providing leisure services because children–their traditional service population–are decreasing in numbers. They will have to refocus services on the elderly, or the older population will vote down any tax requests for recreation.

PROFESSIONAL IMAGE

Unless the academic world catches up to present and future changes, those entering leisure service professions will be ill-prepared to deliver needed services. Professionals must be trained to work in a variety of nontraditional areas.

With the increase in special populations and new life-styles, training will be needed in therapeutic recreation techniques and in the leisure service needs of these groups.

A growing understanding and respect for the leisure service professional will be gained, as the profession upgrades its image and the public begins to understand the critical need for leisure services.

Work, Health, and Recreation: Aspects of the Total Person

Michael K. Bartalos

A lawyer in upstate New York by the name of Lewis Henry Morgan developed an interest in the local Iroquois Indians and spent much of his spare time studying them. The several books he wrote firmly established him as a key figure in the development of anthropology (Barnouw 1971). For an Iowa physician, Dr. Keith O. Garner, diversion means riding and maintaining his drag-racing car. His devotion to this sport is indicated by the five world drag-racing speed records, 14 national race championships, and 140 regional championships he has won (Baum 1987). Thomas Edward Lawrence, better known as "Lawrence of Arabia," loved to listen to the music of Mozart and Beethoven, and between spells of writing, raced his motorcycle through the countryside. He died during one of these rides in 1935 (Cruickshank 1988). Recreational activity for the surgeon Dr. Lazlo Tauber consisted of building and trading in real estate. According to Forbes (1987), this part-time activity helped him to accumulate well over $450 million since his emigration from Hungary to the United States in 1947. Dr. Tauber still practices medicine and functions as chief of surgery in a hospital.

These examples help to illustrate the variety of interests one can pursue as a hobby, as a recreational activity. While such activities can lead to fame or fortune, these are by no means their primary purposes.

Michael K. Bartalos, MD, is Assistant Professor of Clinical Pediatrics, College of Physicians and Surgeons, Columbia University, New York, NY, and Director of the Institute for Genetic Medicine, New York, NY.

7

ASSUMPTIONS

The following discussion is based on the premises of individuality (everybody is unique) and interaction, leading in time to constant change and interconnectedness. Change is a response to environmental stimuli; it is achieved through an adjustive process which is a matter of self-regulation employing the use of feedback. Interconnectedness is the outcome of perpetual interaction between two or more interacting individuals. Adaptive interrelatedness refers to the functional state of individuals in constant interaction responding to stimuli emanating from the environment and from each other; it encompasses both change and interconnectedness. Living matter is organized into hierarchies whereby smaller aggregates of like entities are included in larger units; there is interaction, or flow of information, taking place horizontally as well as vertically. It is assumed, unless proven otherwise, that present characteristics represented a survival advantage for their original bearers and became universal features during subsequent generations.

LIFE PLAN OF THE INDIVIDUAL

Genetic diversity and exposure to differing environmental influences are responsible for our biological individuality, for our uniqueness. We all have our own perception of the world and of the role we play in it. Our life activities are conducted according to a pattern, our decisions have a certain consistency which mirrors our view of ourselves in relationship to others (Goleman 1987). Some psychologists refer to this as "personal mythology" (Keen 1988), while others speak of a person's "life plan" (Cohen 1985).

In order to formulate and realize a life plan, certain prerequisites must be fulfilled. We can infer the following conditions: (1) a reasonable long life span to allow the realization of our goals, (2) the structural integrity of the body, together with its (3) functional integrity are important, (4) physical stamina is required, as are (5) freedom from pain, (6) a balanced state of mind free of irrational fears, capable of sizing up the environment realistically and responding to it in a rational manner, and (7) a certain level of intelligence. Deficiency in any of these areas can compromise the individual's ability to live according to his life plan.

ADAPTATION TO THE ENVIRONMENT

The survival of the organism in the face of environmental adversities represents coping or adaptation to the environment. Adaptation consists of maintenance of bodily integrity and success in reproduction under ever-changing environmental conditions. From an evolutionary perspective, this means the survival of the individual and the perpetuation of the species. In the case of humans, however, beside survival and reproduction the question of quality also enters into our consideration. For us what matters is not merely the birth of children, but also the conditions into which they will be born. Will they be sick, will they be suffering, will there be societal resources available to them, providing adequate support to develop their potentials fully and thus allow their optimal adaptation to the environment?

There are two basic mechanisms, not mutually exclusive, whereby humans adapt to the environment: (1) by modifying the environment so that its threat is neutralized, i.e., heating a room or a cave and thus eliminating cold, and (2) by modifying bodily functions and structures. Such changes can include bodily adaptation to changing temperatures or immune response to invading bacteria. At times when the innate adaptive abilities of the organisms are not sufficient to cope with environmental challenges, artificial modification by means of medications or surgical interventions might restore the balance.

MENTAL ATTITUDE AS AN ADAPTIVE TOOL

The possession of a proper mental attitude, a mentality of wanting to survive, of willingness to struggle, of not giving up, a quality which in the mental sphere represents vigor, is an important factor in adaptation. It is an attitude that is closely connected to hope; it is fueled by hope.

There appears to be a reciprocal interaction between hope and mental lassitude. Because of mental lassitude we can falsely convince ourselves of the hopelessness of a situation and the meaninglessness of further struggle, and thus we might give up any serious attempts at adaptation. This situation can prevail in depressive states. This represents a maladaptive state based on faulty appraisal of the environment.

Hope is a force that acts as a mobilizer of our adaptive responses in the psychological realm. Hope can spur us to fight even when all odds are against us. Such behavior on the surface appears irrational and consequently might be considered pathological. Overoptimism of this kind, nevertheless, could be the product of an evolutionary selection whereby occasionally unforeseen weaknesses or developments in the environment changed the odds in favor of the uncompromising individual who thereby survived and gained selective advantage.

Overreactions to environmental stimuli are varied and seem to underlie such diverse phenomena as allergic reactions, heroism, and the so-called "violences of passion."

WORK AND LEISURE AS ADAPTIVE ACTIVITIES

From a societal point of view, adaptive activities can be subdivided into work and leisure. We generally consider work as a source of income, which we need to purchase food, clothing, and shelter. In primitive societies, work consists of hunting and food gathering, while in a complex, technically evolved society, it can involve such diverse activities as driving a bus, assisting in the preparation of an income tax return, or programming a computer. Since most of us have to work in order to obtain food and clothing and shelter, and thus to survive, work can be considered a tool of survival, an activity that enables adaptation to the environment. Adaptation to the environment, therefore, can include responses such as the widening of the pupil in darkness, increase in heart rate in response to exertion, sweating in response to heat, as well as getting along with coworkers, coping with rush-hour traffic, and mastering a college curriculum.

Work, for most of us, is an activity performed under external constraints during specific hours at specified locations involving the performance of specified tasks. As such it demands both physical and mental effort. Work is a consuming activity and needs to be interrupted by periods of rest. Rest, along with recreation, is part of our adaptive activities. We would not be able to work for any significant length of time without periods of rest and recreative activities.

STRESS AS AN ADAPTIVE MECHANISM

An organism that is well-adapted to the environment is characterized by physical and mental well-being. Such a state is best maintained if the adaptive capabilities of the organism are not strained close to the limit. In a well-balanced adaptive state, environmental demands are easily handled by genetically determined response mechanisms, and such mechanisms are maintained in a well-functioning state by a proper choice and blend of work, rest, and recreation. Most of the body's adaptive responses take place without our awareness.

When we speak of a stress reaction, we are referring to a state of the organism where coping is not effortless, where extra efforts are being made to adapt, and where such efforts can force their way into our consciousness. The awareness of a stressful situation might have an evolutionary origin. It can have a survival value by summoning conscious effort to alter a threatening situation. Such a conscious effort may consist of active avoidance of the stressor or increased adaptive effort by the organism. Adaptive efforts can range from changed leisure activities through behavior modification and transcendental meditation, to taking medication.

COMPONENTS OF ADAPTATION

It seems to me that we can construct a scheme that illustrates the interplay between people and their activities while coping with environmental challenges. Such a scheme would have to take into account the complementarity and interrelationship between physical well-being and mental well-being on the one hand, and work and leisure activities on the other. At the same time, we should not forget that people are social creatures and that interpersonal interactions are taking place at all times.

Studies conducted on patients revealed that their key quality of life concerns could be grouped under the following headings: (1) interpersonal relations (marriage, family, friends), (2) sexual adjustment, (3) work functions, (4) leisure activities, and (5) physical and emotional symptoms (pain, anxiety) (Cohen-Cole 1985). Since sexual activity is part of interpersonal relations, these concern areas correspond rather closely to components of our above-proposed scheme of adaptive interrelatedness.

BENEFITS OF RECREATIONAL ACTIVITIES

An examination of the possible benefits of recreational activities reveals that practically all the functions enumerated earlier as necessary for the successful adaptation of the organism to the environment are improved by some recreational activity.

Let us consider some recreational activities and their derived benefits. Regular exercise can extend life expectancy, restore functional integrity of the body, and increase vigor. Skills of various kinds can be sharpened by activities such as practicing on a musical instrument, playing bridge or baseball, or engaging in target shooting. Pain can be relieved by exercising affected body parts and by diverting attention through activities which engage the individual. Other benefits of recreation include confidence building, tension relief, reduction of depression and promotion of mental alertness—these are benefits that can help us to change our "frame of mind." Since recreational activities promote interaction with other than work-related contacts and family members, such interactions promote relatedness in an informal and relatively stress-free environment. If one's recreational activity is acting or reciting poetry, role playing and enacting are the derived benefits with applicability to real job situations. This list could be extended. The above-named examples, however, should suffice to illustrate the many benefits one can derive from properly chosen recreational activities.

CHOICE OF RECREATIONAL ACTIVITIES

What guides do we have in the selection of appropriate recreational activities?

Need is one. Does the individual need an activity which is performed in quiet solitude or does s/he need the galvanizing effect of a noisy company? Is there a need for vigorous physical exercise or is there a need to fill an emotional void by such activities as coaching or tutoring children or helping the infirm?

Age of the individual is a factor to be considered. Recreational activities that are suitable both physically and mentally for a young person might not suit somebody who is in retirement. Playing golf may be more appealing to the latter, while the former may prefer to play baseball; tennis might be enjoyed by both if played with appropriate partners.

The health status of the individual is an important factor in the decision. The recreational activities of healthy individuals might be labelled as preventive recreation, while recreation during a recovery period from illness can be called therapeutic recreation or recreational therapy. Therapeutic recreation will often differ from preventive recreation and might differ from post-recovery or rehabilitative recreation.

A limiting factor not to be ignored is the availability of resources. One is able to choose only among those possibilities which are given. Once we decide on the type of recreational activity that will likely fill the person's need, narrow down the choices to those that are appropriate for age and health status, and ascertain that the resources are available and affordable to the person, the final criterion is that the activity should be *enjoyable.*

If a person does not find a recreational activity enjoyable, the whole purpose of the activity is defeated. In such cases the activity will become another chore and it will increase the burden of daily existence instead of lightening it.

CONCLUSION

The evaluation of the sources of a patient's difficulties in adaptation to the environment and finding the right recreational activities based on rational consideration can be a complex task. Our goal is the promotion of an optimal balance between the individual patient and his or her environment by every means possible. While we know that our efforts are doomed to eventual failure–since we are all mortal–we consider it our obligation to bargain for time, to fill life with meaningful experiences, and allow it to be lived productively, with dignity and joy. Well-chosen recreational activities are a means to this end.

REFERENCES

Barnouw, V. 1971. *An Introduction to Anthropology, Vol. 2: Ethnology.* Homewood, IL: Dorsey Press.

Baum, A.Z. 1987. "Is This the World's Fastest Doctor?" *Medical Economics,* pp. 144-153.

Cohen, C. 1985. "Philosophical Reflections on the Impact of Coronary Artery Surgery: Patients' Quality of Life." *Quality of Life and Cardiovascular Care,* May-June, pp. 209-214.

Cohen-Cole, S.A. 1985. "Interviewing the Cardiac Patient: A Practical Guide for Assessing Quality of Life." *Quality of Life and Cardiovascular Care,* November-December, pp. 7-12.

Cruickshank, I. 1988. "Lawrence of England." *M.D.,* August, pp. 98-105.

Forbes. 1987. "The Richest People in America." *Forbes Special Edition,* October, p. 180.

Goleman, D. 1987. "Leading Psychologist Expands the Boundaries." *The New York Times,* October 20, pp. C1, C13.

Keen, S. 1988. "Personal Myths Guide Daily Life." *Psychology Today,* December, pp. 43-47.

Balancing Changing Health Care Needs with the Shortage of Quality Health Care Professionals: Implications for Therapeutic Recreation

Peg Connolly

The focus of this volume is on enhancing the quality of life through recreation, with an emphasis on the psychosocial issues confronting the life-threatened patient, family, staff, and community. Before proceeding with my own area of emphasis, the dilemma of balancing expanded health care needs with the shortage of qualified personnel in the field of therapeutic recreation, I would like to address the focus of the volume specifically.

This issue has long been of concern to many in our field. Enhancing the quality of life of those we serve has been the cornerstone of our profession, but it is an effort that has not often been well-received by those outside our professional ranks. In a society such as ours, which is so focused on life, life-saving efforts, and the utility of human activity, there appears to be a sort of abandonment of individuals faced with life-threatening illnesses and conditions. Once the need for medical intervention to save life is considered ineffective, we somehow seem to be at a loss to offer much else to patients, families, and friends. For, without the illusion of unlimited life, or at least, of life without known limits, there seems to be a question of the value of the life at hand regardless of any projected idea of the length of that life. Whether or not our life is threatened by an illness or condition that potentially shortens our expected life

Peg Connolly, PhD, CTRS, is Executive Director, National Council for Therapeutic Recreation Certification, Spring Valley, NY.

span, I do not believe we should be faced with the decision to lessen the quality of that life.

Each day as we learn more of the means to treat and extend human life, we also face the realities of new illnesses and conditions that threaten life despite the technological advances we have made. In addition, we sometimes have the capability of extending life functions while questions arise regarding the quality of the life that remains. Enhancing quality of life may become more acceptable as a goal of treatment in the future when we continue to accumulate examples of the shortcomings, as well as the benefits, of technology in the struggle to preserve life.

In the profession of therapeutic recreation, we have traditionally been concerned with the quality and potential of human life, despite the diagnostic implications of an illness or the less than favorable outlook of any human condition. Our focus has been on the ability, rather than the disability, of the individual. And through this focus on ability, we have often sought to aid individuals in their recovery and/or adjustment by emphasizing their control over their own life, beginning with their control of their ability to experience and enjoy life to the greatest extent possible. While our professional values have been focused on this quality of life perspective, our employment positions and our funding sources for service delivery have at times placed us at odds with our primary concerns. At times, our concern for quality of life has not been considered essential or necessary for effective and efficient medical treatment, and our services are often the first to be cut in times of cost containment.

However, it has not only been the medical and health care business community which has underestimated the value of our services. The patient and family have at times rejected the need for quality of life services. Somehow, the medical community, the patient, the family, and society at large must come together to reexamine the worth and value of addressing quality of life issues in the treatment and care of illnesses and social conditions. We in the field of therapeutic recreation certainly have interventions and approaches that directly address the development of quality of life concerns via recreation. But, first, there must be some perceived value attached to this area of health and human service. There must be some acceptance of the need and desire to receive this type of care.

THE PROFESSION OF THERAPEUTIC RECREATION

Such descriptors as "the profession in transition," or "the emerging profession" applied to therapeutic recreation, imply the dynamics of growth, development, and change. Certainly, this change suggests both a broadened view of people served, and a heightened awareness of our needs in professional growth and development.

We in this field have struggled toward defining our profession and our services, as neither have often been well understood within the mainstream of health care and human services. There have been ongoing debates in our field as to whether the strength of our services lies in the use of recreation activity as a means to an end, or as an end in itself. On one side, those committed to the treatment modality have argued that recreation activity is best used as a therapeutic modality to accomplish treatment goals. On the other side, those committed to the value of recreation as a natural component of human functioning have claimed that recreation is therapeutic in its own right and an end in itself that leads to positive human benefits for those involved.

I dare say these debates on the "ultimate purpose and value" of our service will continue throughout our future as they have through the last 30 to 40 years. These debates show evidence of a concern for bringing meaning to, and defining the potential of, our profession. What underlies both or any of the other perspectives on the purpose and nature of therapeutic recreation services has been a definitive focus on the strengths and needs of the individual service recipient and the fact that the recipient, first and foremost, has the right to the highest quality of life, given his or her illness or condition. Leisure and recreation are seen as necessary components of human functioning and as potential enhancers of the individual's quality of life.

My hope for our profession is that we continue to emphasize our concerns for the persons receiving our services, and that we recognize that our struggle for professional identity and acceptance is a means of continually evaluating our worth as a profession, and defining areas which we, as the professional collective, wish to improve. We will probably never have 100 percent agreement among ourselves as to a single purpose, function, and outcome for our field. However, I believe we need not be immobilized by our debates. We must continue to move forward for the sake of our ideals of quality of care for our clients, our constituencies, and ourselves as professionals.

SHORTAGE OF QUALIFIED HEALTH CARE PROFESSIONALS

We and other health care/human service professions face some incredible dilemmas in the next two decades. We will experience an increase in health care opportunities in our country through the year 2000. The United States Bureau of Labor Statistics projects that there will be a three percent growth in health services and a two percent growth in social services between 1985 and 2000. While the fastest employment growth will be in business, health services will provide as many or more jobs than the business sector. In 1986, there were 7.6 million jobs in health services, and by the year 2000 that number is expected to grow to over 10 million jobs.

Of all health service jobs, those in hospitals will remain high at 42 percent, and provide two of five jobs in the health service arena. In 1988 alone, over 200,000 positions were added in hospitals in the United States. The next highest growing areas will be physician offices and nursing homes. It is important to note here that the Bureau of Labor Statistics is addressing health care needs and jobs in terms of traditional treatment and service means. This does not begin to take into account the numbers of individuals who may desire or require services in their homes that may not involve active medical treatment but may be necessary, as active medical services are no longer indicated while the effects of their illnesses and conditions continue to be problematic to their quality of life. If these potential needs could be analyzed, the numbers of health and human service professionals needed for the future would be much higher than what projections now indicate.

At the same time that we will experience more opportunities for our field, there is a dramatic shortage of personnel to fill these increased health care positions in all health service professions. Part of this can be explained by our population shift, which indicates for the first time a reduction in the 16-24 year-old labor force. Traditionally, this age group has filled many entry-level positions. However, because of low birth rates in the 1960s, we will not see an increase in this age group for the labor force until the baby-boomers' children come into the 16-24 age bracket. So who will fill these entry-level positions that are so essential to health care? It is projected that all professions must reexamine their entry-level work force. Our future work force will include more women and members of minority groups. However, it will be our responsibility to recruit and train these individuals for access to our field.

While we have not conducted a comprehensive supply/demand study of the profession of therapeutic recreation to date, the United States Department of Labor Statistics estimates that there were approximately 29,000 employment positions in recreation therapy as of 1986. It is projected that positions in our field will increase by 20 percent by the year 2000. The field is healthy, therefore, in the labor and occupational outlook, but how will we fill these employment needs? Current information from professionals in the field indicates that we are unable to fill present positions with qualified personnel. Additional information from our educators indicates that student enrollments are declining in some parts of the country. Certainly, I have not spoken to many educators who have difficulty reporting a 90-95 percent placement rate for their graduates.

At this time of transition in our field, we must not only look at critical issues and professional tradition, but we must also examine how we will provide our services in the future. It is time to take a critical look at our current values concerning personnel and professional service delivery. The shortage of qualified therapeutic recreation personnel in this country is significant and, at the same time, there seems to be an increased demand for our services as evidenced by increased job opportunities in the field. Related to this concern with shortages is the reduced pool of therapeutic recreation educators to fill academic positions. Therefore, we will also need a concerted effort to recruit the education personnel necessary to staff training programs in the near future. These are very critical issues facing our profession and its future.

I believe it is time to examine our service provision practices and to consider a greater training of and employment of paraprofessional employees working under the direction of professional staff. It is time to stop our lip-service regarding increased opportunities for and involvement of minority group members and to actively create educational opportunities that allow the nontraditional entry-level person the opportunity to complete training and education requirements while being actively employed in service delivery at the paraprofessional level. We must broaden our concepts of the ideal staffing structure. We must redefine the roles and responsibilities of the therapeutic recreation practitioner, indicating the nature of responsibility that must be provided by a fully qualified professional, and that which may be provided by paraprofessional and technician level staff under the supervision of a fully qualified professional.

Considering the critical demands facing our field for greater levels of sophistication in service delivery, the need for more precise documentation of effective intervention, the greater requirements for employing sound methods of research and evaluation to justify service efficacy, it is sometimes frustrating to imagine a lesser reliance on professional level personnel and a greater use of extender or assistant staff who develop their skills through on-the-job training and certification programs. Truly, there are those in our field who believe the baccalaureate degree cannot prepare professionals with adequate skills for the high demands of clinical health care today, and they cry out for the advanced clinician who enters the field after graduate study. Perhaps we need not give up our desires for more highly trained professionals, but we must not be so shortsighted as to close off any opportunities for access to our field when the need for new personnel is so dramatic. It will be more to our advantage to clarify the roles and responsibilities of various levels of therapeutic recreation personnel, citing legitimate qualifications in tune with various levels of responsibilities, than to limit access. Our main concern should remain with the needs of the patients and clients whom we serve. There are certainly ways to ensure quality care based on client needs and to delineate personnel roles and privileges in relation to these needs, rather than to artificially close our ranks at this time.

At the same time as we need to define our personnel roles with an open focus on providing needed services, we must be fully cognizant of the fact that the labor supply for entry-level personnel willing to enter educational programs in the health care professions is at the lowest level ever in our society. We must be creative in our efforts to recruit and develop our own entry-level labor pool who may progress through levels of education throughout their work careers. Further, while we examine these nontraditional methods of personnel use in our field, we must always continue to strive for improved quality of care in our services.

CONCLUSION

We face some dramatic challenges in our future as a profession. We must somehow juggle the increased needs and demands for our services with the fact that we have a reduced supply of personnel available to provide these services. I believe we can look at this stage of our professional development as a transition, and one that we can address in a positive light. I believe we will have the potential to extend ourselves to new areas of service demand and adequately address these critical needs for care while, at the same time, we will be able to address our desperate need for an adequate personnel pool for our field. We will have this potential if we seriously address the concerns today.

Our focus must remain on the quality of life needs and potential of the patients and clients we serve. Our energies may need to be directed to creative and nontraditional methods of educating our future paraprofessional and professional personnel, but our hopes for our profession should remain high.

We have accomplished so much in the past ten years. We have increased understanding of our services, which tend to add quality to the client's life as opposed to merely reducing symptomatology, on which so many others in health care focus. We have accomplished so much in the past few years that it has made us aware of all that remains to be accomplished. And we have not lessened the vigor with which we face the challenge of balancing the needs of our clientele and the demands of our profession.

Each of us has much to contribute to the advancement of this profession. Each of us has a responsibility to be open to the changing demands for our services. Each of us has a responsibility to maintain our focus on the needs of our clients from the humanistic perspective, from the holistic approach, from the point of view of their ultimate potential for the highest quality of life.

ADDITIONAL READING

Connolly, P. 1989. "Foreword." *Issues in Therapeutic Recreation: A Profession in Transition*. D. Compton, Ed. Champaign, IL: Management Learning Laboratories.

U.S. Department of Labor, Bureau of Labor Statistics. 1988-89. *Occupational Outlook Handbook*.

U.S. Department of Labor, Bureau of Labor Statistics. *Projection 2000: Revised Employment, Output, and Demand for the Year 2000*.

Clinical Effectiveness
of Intensive Therapeutic Recreation:
A Multiple Case Study
of Private Practice Intervention

Robin Kunstler
Steven Sokoloff

The provision of therapeutic recreation (TR) services to individuals with disabilities is the mission of the therapeutic recreation profession. These services historically have been offered in institutional settings, to individuals residing there, via group activities and programs. Gunn and Peterson (1978) stated that social interaction in groups has long been regarded as one of the strongest assets in the leisure movement, although it is naive to "cast people together and expect them to emerge miraculously as changed individuals" (p. 94). More recently, the concept of individualized program or treatment planning has emerged as one of the essential elements in therapeutic recreation programming philosophy and approaches. The individual plan is usually implemented in group situations, however, due to limitations and constraints of staffing, funding, available time, and lack of confidence in professional skills. MacMahon (1979) cited problems of funding, managerial restraints, lack of consumer choice, and limited resources as inherent in public vocational rehabilitation services as well. Understandably, individual services are considered more effective, due to a greater timeliness and personalization, than group services (Matkin 1980).

Robin Kunstler, REd, is Coordinator, Recreation Department, Lehman College of CUNY, Bronx, NY. Steven Sokoloff, MED, is Director, Recreational Associates, New York, NY.

Clinicians also experience frustration over recidivism of rehabilitation and psychiatric clients who are unable to transfer their clinical gains to the home and community settings. Rehabilitation requires intensive use of skilled personnel who are able to devote substantial amounts of time and thought to each case (Matkin 1980b). Institutional programs are rarely able to provide follow-up services after discharge. Therefore, "dropping out" of treatment is the most common mode of termination in community mental health centers, and is a pervasive problem for the fields of rehabilitation, psychotherapy, and health care (Buhrmaster et al. 1982).

One possible solution may be offered by the TR professional in private practice. Private practice or private for-profit TR service refers to the individual TR practitioner who has developed her/his own business, alone or in partnership, to provide individual or group TR services. This has come about in response to the current economic trend toward entrepreneurship as well as to practitioners' desires for expanded outlets for their increasingly sophisticated professional skills. As qualifications and capabilities of personnel have increased, so has frustration with the traditional health care setting and a search for new areas of innovation.

Many agencies have hired TR consultants to provide staff training, program development, and documentation as demands for accountability and quality assurance have reached the TR programs. In addition, the clientele served by health care systems in general has widened, to include the frail elderly, persons with head injuries, substance abusers, and people with AIDS, requiring new treatment philosophies and approaches. The TR practitioner is therefore providing services outside of the institutional setting. This has led to the evolution of the role of TR consultant to TR specialist in private practice, who may be more successful with given clients due to the more intensive, specialized one-to-one treatment that cannot be provided in the traditional setting.

The present study was a preliminary attempt to investigate the effectiveness of TR services provided by a private practitioner to clients for whom traditional treatment was not successful. A multiple case study method was used. The case study method asks explanatory questions of "how" and "why." It requires no control over behavioral events and focuses on contemporary events. Using direct observation and systematic interviewing, its results are generalizable to theories, not to populations. This approach has been used to study the effects and values of recreation, community integration, skill acquisition, and teaching methods/strategies. It can also provide a detailed description of an individual in order to assess program efforts in terms of staff activities, and the extent to which their activities are directly related to the achievement of program objectives (Theobald 1979).

The literal replication approach to multiple case studies was used in the present investigation. Each individual case study consists of a "whole" study, in which convergent evidence is sought, with similar results (a literal replication) predicted at the outset of the investigation (Yin 1984). In the multiple case report, single cases are not presented, but rather a synthesis of different factors using examples from each case.

In the present study, five cases are discussed. Sokoloff, the director of Recreational Associates (R.A.), provided private, individualized TR services to five clients referred to him after traditional treatment approaches had failed to produce adequate gains. A very brief synopsis of each case is provided below, following a summary of the cases. As shown, all five received hospital care and some outpatient treatment, usually physical therapy.

Subjects were four males, ages 20, 26, 32 and 46, and a female, 48 years old. The 46-year-old male was a victim of heart attack with brain injury; the other four suffered catastrophic injuries from motor vehicle accidents. All five had received physical and occupational therapy for periods ranging from three months to three years prior to referral to R.A. All five had ambulation impairments, three requiring a cane, crutches, or braces. Three suffered cognitive deficits including memory loss; three had chronic pain. Other problems included depression, sleeplessness, and post-traumatic stress. After an initial assessment of leisure pursuits, lifestyle, health style and wellness, goals were set that included improving physical functioning and cognitive skills, developing new interests, increasing self-confidence and independence, and decreasing depression. The treatment program typically included corrective exercise and adaptive sports three to five days per week, three to five hours per day. Clients participated in adapted swimming, walking programs, and

Nautilus and Universal weight training. In two cases, adapted electronic games and crafts were utilized once a week to improve cognitive skills such as concentration and coordination, and fine motor skills, and to expand leisure interests. Community reorientation on available services, programs, and transportation for people with disabilities was provided to increase independence. Weekly leisure counseling sessions focused on development of leisure interests, educational goals and choices, and ways to earn income through part-time work. Treatment programs were designed for 6 to 36 months duration.

Improvements were noted in 2 to 25 months. In all cases ambulation improved to walking longer distances, some without mobility aids. Physical condition, cognition, and social interaction improved. Two who began attending community college also earned income through part-time positions in sales and catering. Four developed leisure interests such as jogging, crafts, and cooking. One became continent.

In two cases insurance coverage became an issue. After agreeing to cover treatment costs, the insurance company reneged after four months. The client maintained gains but made no further improvement without continuing treatment. In one case, (case #5), it took three years from referral of the client to the insurance company's approval of payments. During this period, the client was hospitalized numerous times. Coverage was finally approved for a 60-day trial. The insurance company acknowledged that gains were made (ability to walk one block improved to nine blocks) but refused to approve further services. The client regressed to a status below that at the onset of treatment, including full wheelchair use and social withdrawal.

Client #1 was a 20-year-old male, injured in an automobile accident, with a diagnosis of head trauma, fractures of the right arm and leg. He received outpatient occupational therapy and physical therapy once a week for one year, at which time he still could not use his right arm, had a brace on his right leg, and suffered short-term memory loss.

Goals were set to improve strength and endurance, reduce loss of kinesthetic awareness, reduce depression and inactivity, increase self-confidence, and develop new interests and realistic life goals.

After six months of R.A. treatment, including exercises and swimming, the leg brace was removed and the client was able to walk up to one mile without resting. He developed interests in model building and jogging, entered community college, and began selling Amway products part-time.

Client #2, a 46-year-old male bartender, runner, and gourmet cook, had a heart attack while jogging, fell, and suffered a brain concussion. After several months of outpatient physical therapy, the client walked with a cane, was incontinent, required assistance with self-care, and was irritable and confused. Goals included reducing anger and depression and increasing strength, endurance, cognitive function, self-care and socialization. Following four months of five-times-a-week R.A. exercise, cognitive retraining, community re-orientation, and instruction in self-care, the client's incontinence was reduced to one incident a month; he could stay alone up to four hours and walk independently in his neighborhood. Start of treatment had been delayed one year due to the insurance company's reluctance to pay for treatment.

Client #3, an unemployed 32-year-old male, broke both legs in an automobile accident. Inpatient psychiatric care and occupational and physical therapy were received, followed by two months of outpatient physical therapy. The client walked with crutches, experiencing lower back pain, depression and nightmares. Family interaction was tense and the client mostly watched television, read, and slept. Goals included improving physical ability, self-image and self-confidence; reducing depression; and developing new interests. After two years of R.A. treatment, the client relocated, developed social and leisure skills, and received instruction in home-based income-producing activity. He no longer required use of a crutch.

Client #4, a 48-year-old female, experienced chronic pain from injuries sustained in an automobile accident, in addition to stress and tension. She received inpatient and outpatient physical therapy and could walk with a cane. She was also receiving psychiatric care. Shortly before her accident she had moved to a new state and had become socially isolated. The client desired to return to school, to work, and to leisure pursuits. After twelve months of R.A. treatment, she could walk and bicycle (a former interest) 3.6 miles with two stops. She entered community college in a career training program, developed craft and cooking hobbies, and eventually started a home business.

Client #5, a 25-year-old male, was also catastrophically injured in an automobile accident. He had post-traumatic stress disorder, leg and back pain, shoulder and knee injuries, and was a paranoid schizophrenic. He received three years of extensive treatment during numerous hospitalizations, including physical and occupational therapy, chiropractic and acupuncture treatment. He spent most of his time in bed, angry, depressed, and withdrawn. He could walk one block using a cane and stopping for rest periods. He could not use his right arm. A two-to-three year, five-days-per-week treatment program was designed by R.A., including extensive exercise. His walking ability improved to nine blocks after two months. The client began to play board and electronic games and read books and magazines. Due to insurance payment problems, services were discontinued, and the client regressed to full wheelchair use and social withdrawal.

As described in these cases, the hospital and outpatient treatment and care received did not begin to address the multitude of physical and emotional problems brought on by these clients' catastrophic injuries. One-to-one treatment, by its nature and as provided by R.A., is intensive and tailored to the specific needs and interests of clients. Results showed that all five clients improved in areas of physical condition, cognitive skills, leisure interests, and mood. When programs did not run full course due to payment problems, clients either did not show further improvement or regressed. Why did TR succeed where other treatments did not? Two factors may explain this. One is the intensity of treatment: three to five days per week for three to four hours per day. With this type of intensive, individualized service, it is conceivable that other therapies could also succeed. But could a person tolerate that much treatment without the qualities of recreation to make it not only bearable, but pleasurable? Couple this with the second factor, the holistic approach of TR treatment. TR focuses on physical, cognitive, and emotional functioning in leisure, education, vocational, and community aspects of living. Occupational therapy may also make this claim. However, the emphasis on leisure experience, on fulfilling oneself through one's daily pursuits, may be more potent than focus on restoration of mere daily function. "To what end?" the client may wonder. TR provides a reason.

As the number of clients eligible for rehabilitation-oriented services increases due to deinstitutionalization, increases in the elderly population, increases in life expectancy associated with many diseases and chronic health conditions, and more stress-related and mental health ailments, including substance abuse (Kunstler 1986), funding for services will decrease (Matkin 1980a). It appears that a private practitioner can be useful when he or she can supply services unavailable from employers, inhouse programs, or governmental agencies, or when he or she can act more quickly and economically than any of these other service providers. The private sector could also be utilized to provide specific services to clients on a contractual basis in specialty areas (Matkin 1980b). Perhaps private, individualized TR services can more effectively rehabilitate and restore to functioning clients who have been unsuccessful in traditional treatment, such as victims of catastrophic injury, including damage to the brain and/or spinal cord, and those with depression. Reimbursement for these services may then be forthcoming as third-party payers acknowledge the success and the cost-effectiveness, not to mention the moral obligation, of returning a client to maximal lifestyle functioning. Future research should investigate further the efficacy of these services and compare their cost to that of other forms of treatment.

REFERENCES

Buhrmaster, D., J. Hartman, P. Menefee, E. M. Shores, and R. W. Rogers. 1982. "Clients' Reasons for Dropping out of Rehabilitation Center." *Psychological Reports* 51: 1307-1316.

Gunn, S. and C. Peterson. 1978. *Therapeutic Recreation Program Design.* Englewood Cliffs, N.J.: Prentice-Hall, Inc.

Kunstler, R. 1986. "Current Health Problems, Trends in Health Care and Demand for Recreation and Leisure Services Personnel." *Visions in Leisure and Business* 5 (1 and 2): 7-12.

MacMahon, B. T. 1979. "Private Sector Rehabilitation: Benefits, Dangers and Implications for Education." *Journal of Rehabilitation* 3:56-59.

Matkin, R. E. 1980a. "Public/Private Rehabilitation During Recession." *Journal of Rehabilitation,* 4:58-61.

Matkin, R.E., 1980b. "The Rehabilitation Counselor in Private Practice: Perspectives for Education and Preparation." *Journal of Rehabilitation* 3:60-62.

Theobald, W. F. 1979. *Evaluation of Recreation and Park Programs*. New York: John Wiley & Sons, Inc.

Yin, R. K. 1984. *Case Study Research: Design and Methods*. Beverly Hills: Sage Publications.

Quality of Living Until Death: A Fusion of Death Awareness into Therapeutic Recreation-Leisure Education

Carol Stensrud

Death is the one fact of my life which is not relative but absolute, and my awareness of this gives my existence and what I do each hour an absolute quality. (Rollo 1958, p. 49)

This article will explore the linkage of death awareness to the therapeutic recreation profession. More specifically, it will address the relationship of leisure education and death awareness. The potential integration of the two concepts will be explored related to settings that serve individuals and families at risk–those faced with potentially terminal, life-threatening situations.

A girl named Jean, only 14, though quite tall and perhaps mature for her age, became a nurse's aide, following the path of her mother who was a registered geriatric nurse. The first day on the job the girl was given her assignment. "Here is your wing," she was informed. In actuality, she was neither "informed" nor qualified for this assignment.

Jean went forth to do the best she could, working with individuals who were institutionalized, elderly, ill, and often

Carol Stensrud, PhD, is Associate Professor, Department of Recreation and Leisure Studies, School of Health & Human Services, California State University at Sacramento, Sacramento, CA.

This article is a revision of an article that was previously published in *Leisure Information Quarterly,* Volume 18(1), 1991-92, pp. 4-7.

frail. One of the patients was a woman, Ann, with cancer, weighing less than 80 pounds and in extreme pain. She lay behind a drawn curtain that separated her from her roommate, who was drowsing in front of the television set. When Jean greeted Ann, the response was a low moan.

Jean touched her body in a gesture of comfort and was shocked to find her all bones. She pulled back the sheets to view a decubitus ulcer that nearly covered Ann's entire back. Carefully she performed a peroxide procedure. Ann was uncomfortable. Jean withdrew.

Very soon after this, Ann died. Jean's emotions ran wild. Her first thought was that she had killed her. "What an incompetent I am. I wasn't prepared." Panic. Guilt.

Her second thoughts suggested that all might have been "well and good." Ann was not really living. She was in extreme mental and physical pain, a bare shadow of her true being, living only a fragment of the quality of life she would want. Better to die than live a life of pain and loneliness, of diminished physical and cognitive ability.

While struggling with these thoughts, Jean was further shocked by the secretive response to Ann's death. In a dread silence, Ann was whisked off quickly to the morgue, all room doors closed so that no one could see her exit. Her roommate was informed that Ann had gone for a visit to the hospital. The staff who cared for her for years were given no more explanation than that she had "expired." Even more disturbingly, no one had offered Ann a chance to express her feelings before she died. Her family members were given no opportunity to say goodbyes, make acknowledgments, relate to one another and deal with the issues of death and dying.

A few years later, Jean faced her own personal near death experience through an operable cancer. Facing potential early death, she clarified the aim of her life, which was not to work and work simply to accumulate. She felt that she should do and give and love. She became a recreation therapist.

Jean continues to ponder the question: How do we infuse death awareness into leisure services and specifically into therapeutic recreation services? And more importantly, *why* do we do this?

THE "WHY" OF DEATH AWARENESS

Kundera's recently acclaimed novel, *The Unbearable Lightness of Being* (1984), offers a look at the force that living with an awareness of death provides: "The heavier the burden the closer our lives come to the earth, and the more real and truthful they become" (p. 5).

Death, or rather dying, is perceived as a heavy burden that often weights us down. This can be interpreted positively. Death puts us solidly on the ground, encouraging us, compelling us to move with direction and concentration on our living. In denying death as a reality, we deny ourselves the heaviness that allows us to walk forward in a real and truthful manner.

Conversely, denying death denies us the opportunity for lightness. Janis Joplin sang, "Freedom is just another word for nothing left to lose." Only when we face our life's end, nothing left to lose, do we begin to gain a sense of freedom. With this sense of freedom we are released from the everyday, the mundane, and the inane. We are offered a chance to stop protecting, saving, living for the morrow. What is there to lose ultimately? Yourself. Once accepted as a reality, we are free to go and do and be light.

Realization of death holds mixed blessings. Death offers us elements of heaviness that push us down and ground us and allow us to become directed towards the important elements in our lives, rather than just floating aimlessly. Death awareness allows us to be light. It allows us to fly above the foolishness of the perceived burdens and get on with flying like an eagle. Becoming aware of death from a personal perspective becomes an important life directional–the sign in the road. Contemplating dying becomes one of the strongest influences in living.

SETTINGS AND POPULATIONS ADDRESSED

All individuals face death, some perceivably but not necessarily before others. For the purpose of this chapter, the focus will be on those populations viewed as terminally ill. Family, clients, and staff in diverse settings are within heart beats of death. Settings include those serving patients with cancer, heart disease, stroke, multiple sclerosis, muscular dystrophy, head trauma, AIDS and AIDS-related syndromes, leukemia, kidney and liver diseases, substance abuse, and mental illnesses. The list of service settings for persons with potentially life-threatening conditions is growing.

Each of these settings and each individual served there needs to be allowed the opportunity to utilize death as a positive life force, one contributing to quality living. All concerned–patients, families, staff–need to be provided a nonthreatening arena to explore and express the following themes: personal values, current life goals, unfinished business of life, attitudes toward life's end, grief and bereavement, death-related emotions.

It is through the viewing and expression of whatever thoughts and emotions are engendered by these themes that we are allowed opportunities for growth that are otherwise suppressed (Lofland 1978). All of these themes allow for awareness and new perspectives on death, dying and living.

VALUES OF DEATH AWARENESS

The values of death awareness have been addressed by many authors (Green and Irish 1971; Lifton and Olson 1976; Worden and Proctor 1976; Kübler-Ross 1975; Young 1984; Cutter 1974). All of them point to the summation or culminating value of death awareness and its main contribution to living–the gift of love. When the reality of dying is near, we have no time to waste in behaviors that reflect casualness, thoughtlessness or selfishness. Thus death awareness becomes the basis for our humanity, our quality of living.

Scott and Brewer (1971) summarize the salutary consequences of death awareness. They find that individuals achieve integrity and consistency with their own principles, knowing that they have no later negotiations guaranteed. No false threat or coercion can sway them. They achieve honesty, no longer practicing the self-deception that characterizes those who imagine they have a guaranteed future. Accepting death gives them the freedom to take charge of their lives. Realization of death leads to strength, a strength which leads to self-fulfillment. A new perspective is found, often with a sweetened appreciation for every aspect of life, even the mundane.

A COMPARISON OF DEATH AWARENESS AND LEISURE EDUCATION

Death awareness has only recently been recognized as a specific area of study. However, clergy, poets, and artists have studied it through the ages. It is part of what Lofland (1978) calls the happy death movement–"the sprawling, multistructured assemblage of people engaged in a general social movement attempting to establish a new order of life relative to death" (p. 74). This new order of life is one fuller and richer in respect to the values previously discussed. Thus, the happy death movement can also be viewed as a happy life movement.

Death awareness is essentially confronting one's own death and developing resources for encountering the death of others (Worden and Proctor 1976). Personal awareness of death-related values, beliefs, attitudes, orientations, and experiences are central subjects of death awareness. The focus is on identifying and expressing feelings, attitudes, and perceptions of death. In addition, these expressions are viewed with respect to how they affect life fulfillment. Death awareness differs from death education, which may encompass a personal perspective but primarily focuses on sociological, ethical, historical, and cultural perspectives of death and dying.

The processes utilized in death awareness are explorative, open-ended, nonjudgmental. Discussion, value clarification exercises, role playing, poetry, music, pictures, and other creative means are utilized to assist people to gain access to their feelings about death and dying.

Death awareness programs take many formats; individual, group, short term, long term. They are provided by many types of persons: lay persons, physicians, psychiatrists, counselors, nurses, all types of caring professionals, including recreation therapists. The qualifications include a sincere interest, preparation and training.

THE LEISURE LINK

Leisure education has numerous definitions. One of the more commonly accepted is "the broad category of services that focuses on the development and acquisition of various leisure-related skills, attitudes, and knowledge" (Peterson and Gunn 1984, p. 22). It is a helping process that assists persons in gaining and maintaining a fulfilling leisure lifestyle, contributing to their personal happiness and quality of life.

The process of leisure education is usually provided by a recreation professional, often a recreation therapist, having training in leisure education. The qualifications are similar to those of a death awareness facilitator: sincere interest, and adequate training and preparation on the topic and in basic counseling techniques.

The process of leisure awareness is often similar to that of death awareness. Small group or individual work is done, depending on the client's needs. A variety of creative activities is employed. The outcome of leisure education is ideally a lifestyle that offers each individual the maximum opportunity for quality leisure and a balanced, meaningful life–a life that offers each person a chance to be all that he or she can be. A life open to true leisure is defined by Godbey (1985) as "living in relative freedom from the external compulsive forces of one's culture and physical environment so as to be able to act from internally compelling love, in ways which are personally pleasing, intuitively worthwhile, and provide a basis for faith" (p. 79).

THERAPEUTIC RECREATION
PROFESSIONALS ADDRESS DEATH

The therapeutic recreation professional has a responsibility to address death in order to help people live fully until they die. It is our responsibility as professional recreation therapists to address the sensitive subject of death awareness because we often have the best opportunities to do so. We are frequently called upon to be the confidant of our clients. We connect with their expressive domains and encourage cathartic release of emotions through re-creative activities. We are present at some of the most powerful occasions, when, for example, the magic of the leisure experience can open a person to poignant insights.

In order to assist clients to death awareness, the leisure professional needs to be trained in death awareness. Activities which assist death awareness basically focus on self awareness, and thus fit well into a leisure education program.

LIFELINE ACTIVITY

One activity which is often used to develop death awareness, and can be an important part of a leisure education program, is the lifeline activity. The purpose of this activity is to gain perspective on values, priorities, hopes, disappointments, goals, and realities across the lifespan. The activity consists of making a large drawing centering around a line drawn from birth to death, with significant events marked. Creative materials may be used to illustrate or to symbolize events, feelings, insights. Journeying into the known will include past events. Journeying into the unknown requires anticipating the future, even, perhaps, one's death and its circumstances.

Many variations are possible in this activity. Audiovisual equipment may be used; family groups may share the project; it may serve to stimulate memory and thus facilitate reality orientation.

Through this, and other similar activities, perspectives on death can be gained and shared. Death can be seen as part of life, and this awareness can free clients to live life fully, to be in touch with their own deepest values, to cherish the moments of living which remain.

REFERENCES

Cutter, F. 1974. *Coming to Terms with Death.* Chicago: Nelson-Hall Co.

Godbey, G. 1985. *Leisure in Your Life, 2nd ed.* State College PA: Venture Publishing.

Green, B.R, and Irish, D. 1971. *Death Education, Preparation for Living.* Cambridge, MA: Schenkman Publishing Co.

Kübler-Ross, E. 1975. *Death, the Final Stage of Growth.* Englewood Cliffs, NJ: Prentice-Hall.

Kundera, M. 1984. *The Unbearable Lightness of Being.* New York: Harper & Row.

Lifton, R. and Olson, E. 1976. *Living and Dying.* New York: Praeger Publishers.

Lofland, L. 1978. *The Craft of Dying.* London: Sage Publishers.

Peterson, C. A., and Gunn, S. L. 1984. *Therapeutic Recreation Program Design.* (2nd. ed.). Englewood Cliffs, NJ: Prentice-Hall.

Rollo, M. 1958. *Existence.* New York: Basic Books.

Scott, F. & Brewer, W. 1971. *Confrontations of Death.* Eugene, OR: Center for Gerontology.

Worden, W. & Proctor, W. 1976. *Personal Death Awareness: Breaking Free of Fear to Live a Better Life Now.* Englewood Cliffs, NJ: Prentice-Hall.

Young, V. 1984. *Working with the Dying and Grieving.* Davis, CA: International Dialogue Press.

ADDITIONAL READING

Doyle, F. 1978. *Grief Counseling, A Training Manual.* Walnut Creek: Contra Costa Crisis and Suicide Intervention Service.

Kalish, R. (ed) 1979. *Death, Dying, Transcending.* New York: Baywood Publishing Co.

Loesh, L. and Wheeler, P. 1982. *Principles of Leisure Counseling.* Minneapolis, MN: Educational Media Corp.

McDowell, C.F. 1976. *Leisure Counseling: Selected Lifestyle Processes.* Eugene, OR: Center for Leisure Studies.

Psychosocial Issues Confronting Health Care Professionals Working with People with AIDS

Arnold H. Grossman

The first cases of what we now call Acquired Immune Deficiency Syndrome (AIDS) were identified barely a decade ago in New York and California. As no one then could have predicted the course of events relating to this disease in the intervening years, no one now can with certainty predict the future. As of February 6, 1989, however, 85,290 cases of AIDS were reported to the Centers for Disease Control (CDC) (Diesenhouse 1989); and of these more than 36,000 were alive and in potential need of care and services (Lambert 1989). And as the CDC points out, these cases are only the tip of the iceberg. Many more people have AIDS-related conditions caused by the Human Immunodeficiency Virus (HIV) while others are HIV-infected and are not aware of it. The Federal government estimates about 1 to 1.5 million individuals in the United States are infected with HIV (Lambert 1988).

SOME ASSUMPTIONS

Let us begin with some assumptions about HIV infection and AIDS so that the psychosocial issues confronting therapeutic recreation specialists can be viewed in proper perspective.

Arnold H. Grossman, PhD, CSW, CLP, is Chairman and Professor, Recreation and Leisure Studies, School of Education, Health, Nursing and Arts Professions, New York University, New York, NY.

Let us agree that AIDS is caused by HIV and that it is transmitted by sex contact–vaginal, oral, or anal–with someone who is infected, or by sharing needles and syringes with an infected person. Babies of women who are infected with HIV may be born with the infection because it can be transmitted from the mother to the baby before or during birth.

Let us agree that HIV is not transmitted by casual contact and that it is not transmitted through sweat, tears, or saliva, in spite of the fact that small amounts of HIV have been found in these bodily fluids.

Let us agree that the opportunistic infections associated with HIV are treatable, although AIDS is not curable. And most people who are infected with HIV experience a variety of illnesses and disabling conditions over several years, including those involving the central nervous system, e.g., forgetfulness and dementia.

Let us agree that at this time the large majority of all adults with AIDS are gay or bisexual men or intravenous drug users (IVDUs). They are predominantly between the ages of 20 and 49–an age when most people are not commonly prepared to deal emotionally with a life-threatening disease.

Let us agree that "few other diseases produce as many losses–loss of physical strength, mental acuity, ability to work, self-sufficiency, social roles, income and savings, housing, and the emotional support of loved ones. Often, self-esteem also fades in the wake of such catastrophic losses" (National Institute of Mental Health 1986, p. 1).

BLAMING THE VICTIM

This article will seek to explore the psychosocial issues confronting health care professionals working with people with AIDS, especially therapeutic recreation specialists, in the context of victim blaming and old-fashioned conservative ideologies. According to Ryan (1976), "Blaming the Victim is an ideological process, which is to say that it is a set of ideas and concepts deriving from systematically motivated, but unintended, distortions of reality" (p. 11). Ryan indicates that this process takes place so smoothly it appears to be rational, and he identifies it as follows: First, identify the social problem. Second, study those affected by the problem and discover in what ways they are different from the rest of us as a consequence of deprivation and injustice. Third, define the differences as the cause of the social problem itself. Finally, of course, assign a government bureaucrat to invent a humanitarian action program to correct the differences (p. 8).

In his discussion, Ryan indicates that Blaming the Victim is quite different from what he calls "old-fashioned conservative ideologies. The latter simply dismissed victims as inferior, genetically defective, or morally unfit; the emphasis is on the intrinsic, even hereditary, defect. The former shifts its emphasis to the environmental causation" (p. 7).

The reader may ask what this has to do with psychosocial issues confronting therapeutic recreation specialists working with people with AIDS. I would submit that all professionals working with people with AIDS have to examine these issues relating to the large majority of people with whom they are working, namely, gay and bisexual men, intravenous drug users, and a disproportionate number of members of ethnic and racial minority groups. The first two of these subgroups of the population are still stigmatized by what Ryan calls the old-fashioned conservative ideologies, namely by homophobia, i.e., an unnatural fear of homosexual persons, and a phobia against IVDUs based on the belief that they are inferior, genetically defective, or morally unfit. The latter subgroup, namely racial and ethnic minority group members, have been subjected to the process of victim blaming. As Ryan states, "The racial situation in America is usually acknowledged to be a number one item on the nation's agenda. Despite years of marches, commissions, judicial decisions, and endless legislative remedies, we are confronted with unchanging or even widening racial differences in achievement" (p. 9). We have to learn to reframe our reality, learn not to see simply minorities, but members of minority groups who engage in high-risk behaviors.

The socialization of health care providers in our society, like the socialization of all other individuals, includes the above-mentioned societal views of homosexuals, bisexuals, IVDUs and ethnic and racial minorities. Added to this are the facts that HIV was first identified in gay men and AIDS was called Gay Related Immune

Deficiency (GRID), and that it has spread disproportionately among IVDUs and minority group members. The resulting magnified, internalized, and unfounded prejudices, antilocutions, and discriminatory practices toward these doubly stigmatized individuals provide psychosocial issues and ethical dilemmas for health care professionals who are attempting to provide needed services to clients with a life-threatening disease.

ROLE OF THE THERAPEUTIC RECREATION SPECIALIST

The role of therapeutic recreation specialists in working with people with HIV infection or AIDS is becoming more crucial. As medical interventions with the opportunistic infections associated with HIV infection are becoming more effective, individuals are tending to live longer and are seeking to empower themselves regarding the factors related to their health status. Among these factors are stress reduction, self-expression, relaxation, appropriate nutrition intake, socialization with like-minded individuals, and diversionary recreation activities. It is in these areas that therapeutic recreation specialists have the professional training and expertise. They can develop therapeutic recreation intervention strategies which can assist the individuals to meet not only these expressed needs but those related to feelings of helplessness, reduced self-esteem and physical capacity, emotional and social isolation, and the stressed coping mechanisms associated with the diagnosis of and living with AIDS.

Not only are therapeutic recreation specialists responsible for providing direct clinical services to clients, but they are called upon to provide education, consultation and support to others–families, friends, and lovers, the "worried well" in the gay community and sexual partners of IVDUs, health care professionals who may have engaged in high-risk behaviors or have an occupational risk, volunteers whose lifestyle has been similar to those with AIDS or who have friends who are ill or have died from an HIV-related disease, and policy makers who have an impact on the delivery of services.

Before they can work effectively (or at all) with the above-mentioned groups, therapeutic recreation specialists must sort out, confront, and understand personal and professional responses to psychosocial issues that have a tendency to evolve as one begins working with people with HIV infection and AIDS. These are the issues, feelings, biases, and fears which are examined in the remainder of this article.

PSYCHOSOCIAL ISSUES

HIV infection and AIDS present a human challenge for health care providers that might be as big as the scientific and medical challenges. As a result of their socialization, many therapeutic recreation specialists tend to succumb, consciously or unconsciously, to victim blaming and the old-fashioned conservative ideologies. The result is that they tend to blame persons who have contracted HIV infection or AIDS instead of blaming the virus. Consequently, these become the primary psychosocial issues to which they have to respond. These and other issues will be examined within the conceptual framework of countertransference. "Countertransference refers to those conscious, preconscious, and unconscious responses and feelings of the therapist that can be both a problem and a valuable therapeutic and diagnostic tool" (Dunkel and Hatfield, 1986, p. 115).

Stigmatization of Homosexuals and IVDUs

Society has stigmatized homosexuals and IVDUs as "second class" citizens. It has developed myths about these people to support bigotry, discrimination, and oppression. In relation to homosexuals, this is clearly stated by Delaney and Goldblum (1987):

Homophobia, the irrational fear (and often hatred) of gay people, is deeply imbedded in our culture. Although some consider it a normal and moral state of mind, many psychologists now recognize homophobia, not homosexuality, as a mental disorder. When we as gay people show symptoms of this ugly disease, we call it 'internalized homophobia.' It is widespread in our community, although in a more subtle form than that demonstrated by obvious bigots. (p. 269)

This internalization of the dominant group's perception of one-self creates issues not only for the gay person who is HIV-infected, but also for the health care professional who is heterosexual and is working with the patient, as well as for heterosexual health care providers who have unresolved homosexual feelings.

In a 1985 survey of 237 hospital workers involved in the care of AIDS patients conducted at a major AIDS inpatient-care facility in Massachusetts, Pleck et al. (1988) found that "the strong predictive influence of homophobia on negative attitudes toward AIDS is intuitively plausible. It underscores the reality that how people feel about AIDS is, in large part, a function of how they feel about homosexuality" (p. 53).

Education about homosexuals and IVDUs helps one to learn about the unjustified negative statements and helps one learn to stop "blaming the victims." It is important to remember that the virus does not know who is homosexual, bisexual, heterosexual, or IVDU.

Fear of Death and Dying

Feelings about one's own mortality tend to surface when one works with individuals who have life-threatening diseases. "This is not an uncommon dynamic, particularly among health care providers who place such a high priority on 'beating death' " (Dunkel and Hatfield 1986, p. 115). As HIV has taken a disproportionate toll on younger members of the population, this fear is exacerbated by seeing the untimely deaths of children and people who are in the prime of life. Having experiences with death and learning not to deny the personhood of the one dying can help mitigate this fear.

Powerlessness and Helplessness

These feelings result from the inability to: (1) change the course of the disease, (2) successfully treat a series of opportunistic infec-tions, and (3) save lives. They may also emerge in health care providers who have a knowledge deficit regarding the details of HIV or its related diseases. Health care providers need to attend training and educational programs about HIV and its related diseases and to maintain up-to-date knowledge. They also need to learn that being available, reliable, and empathetic is important to optimal care of persons with HIV-infection or AIDS, even though these fall outside the expectations learned in professional training programs.

Anger and Hostility

These feelings usually emerge in relation to, and are directed toward, three groups, namely, fellow health care providers, family, friends or lovers of persons with AIDS, and the public-at-large and legislators. Fellow health care providers become the targets of anger and hostility because of their insensitivity, acts of discrimination or failure to treat. Family, friends, and lovers may arouse the same feelings for their acts of discrimination and recrimination or abandonment. And, the public-at-large and legislators incite these feelings in response to their verbal or behavioral acts of discrimination or their intent to make laws which invade privacy or propose quarantine. Health care providers need to acknowledge these feelings and give themselves permission to express them appropriately, e.g., through advocacy of more funds and facilities. The provider must be certain not to use the person with AIDS as a political tool to express his or her anger at society.

Frustration

Feelings of frustration arise in relation to the reluctance of governments and individuals to effectively cope with the HIV epidemic. There are insufficient numbers of health care providers willing to treat persons who are HIV-infected or have AIDS; insufficient treatment facilities; insufficient skilled nursing facilities or hospices; insufficient numbers of unrestricted drug studies. In addition, working with a large number of people who are chronically ill and who are time-consuming is extremely frustrating. All of these problems are exacerbated by poor case management. Health care providers must become aware of the sources of the frustration and the resulting anger, and they must make certain that it is not misdirected to the person with AIDS.

Working with Difficult Clients

Sometimes labelled noncompliant or obnoxious clients, these are HIV-infected individuals who either continue to have unsafe sex and refuse to tell their sexual partners, or IVDUs who are manipulative and continue to use drugs overtly or covertly. They are also the individuals with neuropsychiatric complications, individuals who threaten or attempt suicide, and infected pregnant women who refuse an abortion. These clients incite feelings of helplessness, fear, and guilt that result in blaming the victim.

"Anger can be an unconscious attempt to punish, leading to irrational, explosive, and unpredictable behavior on the part of the worker. Anger that serves to distance the worker from the client is a form of self-preservation and serves to protect the worker from experiencing the pain of loss and death. . . . Such countertransference blocks empathy and prevents the therapist from being emotionally available during the stages of client need" (Dunkel and Hatfield 1986, p. 116).

Overidentification with Clients

Health care providers who overidentify with clients, e.g., homosexuals, minority group members, or women with children, lose the ability to be objective. As a result of providers meeting personal needs and fusing personal and professional responsibilities, they invest unrealistic amounts of time and energy in specific clients and perhaps their families. Individuals who are vulnerable are workers who have the same lifestyle or are the same age, or individuals with children of their own who are working with children who have become infected via transfusions or from their mothers.

Guilt

This feeling usually emerges in health care workers who are not infected despite their having participated in high-risk behaviors.

Often described as suffering from "survivor's syndrome," these workers feel guilty in the presence of people with AIDS, especially since they are not able to "save" their lives. Workers who are not able to face their professional responsibility of treating people who are HIV-infected also feel guilty. In the latter case, individual counseling might assist the worker in facing denial of the responsibility and assist other workers in obtaining the training to counteract their lack of readiness.

Need for Professional Omnipotence

Many people who are HIV-infected or have AIDS and are on medication know more about their conditions, the side effects of drugs, and alternative treatments than do the health care providers. Consequently, the professional role and identity of the provider is not always acknowledged. This creates negative feelings in the provider. Coping with these feelings by admitting them helps the provider to maintain objective empathy and provide optimal service to clients.

Fear of the Unknown and Fear of Contagion

In health care providers who have received education and training about HIV and AIDS, and who have worked for a number of years with individuals who are infected, the prevalence of these fears has diminished. There are, however, individuals who believe that we do not know for certain all the exact ways that HIV can be transmitted or all possible methods to alter the disease's course. A typical expression of this is: "Maybe what has been published is everything they know so far about AIDS, but what about the unknown?"

Most health care providers have come to accept the knowledge that has been presented about transmission and infection control procedures. There are still some who have an irrational fear of being contaminated and passing the contamination to family, friends and significant others; and many receive pressure from these individuals to discontinue working with people with AIDS. These fears are exacerbated by the secretive and questionable work of researchers such as Dr. Lo of the Armed Forces Institute of Pathology in Washington. Three years after he announced that he had discovered a new virus among AIDS patients, Dr. Lo published his findings. In his paper, Dr. Lo and his team stated: "We have unequivocally demonstrated the existence of a previously unrecognized virus-like infectious agent in patients with AIDS" (Altman 1989, p. c3). Apparently, Dr. Lo has not provided crucial biological reagents to other researchers so that they can attempt to replicate his findings; consequently, it is difficult to determine if this is an important breakthrough or a scientific quirk.

One has to recognize the rational fear of occupational transmission, e.g., needle-sticks, although the rate of such transmission is infinitesimal. Following the universal precautions for health care providers promulgated by the Centers for Disease Control can realistically protect the provider and minimize this fear.

CONCLUSION

The purpose of this article is to assist therapeutic recreation specialists and other health care providers in exploring the psychosocial issues which emerge in working with people who are HIV-infected or have AIDS within the context of victim-blaming and old-fashioned conservative ideologies. Its main intended outcome is to help professionals to accept the human challenge of working effectively with these individuals. Not only will you be fulfilling a professional mandate, but you will be enhancing your professional competence and helping people who will be more appreciative than you can ever imagine.

REFERENCES

Altman, L. 1989, April 11. "AIDS Finding Piques Curiosity but Scientists Are Wary." *The New York Times* p. C3.

Delaney, M. and Goldblum, P. 1987. *Strategies for Survival: A Gay Men's Health Manual for the Age of AIDS.* New York: St. Martin's Press.

Disenhouse, S. 1989, February 12. "AIDS Lessons Replace Tupperware at Parties." *The New York Times,* p. 54.

Dunkel, J. and Hatfield, S. 1986. "Countertransference Issues in Working with Persons with AIDS." *Social Work,* 31(2): 114-117.

Lambert, B. 1989, February 8. "Changing AIDS Epidemic Highlights Shortcomings in Health Care System." *The New York Times*, p. A1.

National Institute of Mental Health. 1986. *Coping with AIDS: Psychological and Social Considerations in Helping People with HTLV-III Infection*. (DHHS Publication No. ADM 85-1432). Washington, D.C.: U.S. Government Printing Office.

Pleck, J., O'Donnel, L., O'Donnell, C., and Snarey, J. 1988. "AIDS-Phobia, Contact with AIDS, and AIDS-related Job Stress in Hospital Workers." *Journal of Homosexuality*, 15 (3/4), p. 41-54.

Ryan, W. 1986. *Blaming the Victim*. New York: Vintage Press.

Occupational Therapy Intervention
in Recreational Activities
in Acute Care Settings

Ann Burkhardt

Occupational therapy is a profession which is based upon the use of occupation, or purposeful activity, to influence the biological, psychological, and social health of an individual.

We analyze activities to determine the occupational performance components of each activity. Performance components include motor functioning, sensory functioning, visual-perceptual functioning, and cognitive functioning. To clarify, we analyze how the body moves, what the body feels, how the eyes guide the mind to see, and how we think and are able to learn.

Occupational performance is the use of these behaviors in purposeful activities which contribute to self-care, interpersonal relationships, work, or play.

Once we have this baseline understanding of a person's abilities, activities are chosen which combine some or all of these components. The goal is to challenge the individual, while providing him/her with a sense of mastery or control, in order to improve his/her functional ability in any or all of the problem areas which an evaluation defines.

Recreation, unlike self-care or work, implies the concept of play. Occupational therapists distinguish between two aspects of recreation: things done for fun or relaxation, and community or group activities. The choice of an appropriate activity is a challenge for the therapist. One person's work is another person's

Ann Burkhardt, MA, OTR, is Chief Occupational Therapist at Memorial Sloan-Kettering Cancer Center, New York, NY.

51

play. Therefore, the recreational activity of choice and the time invested in recreational participation will vary from individual to individual.

Recreational activities should provide potential for enjoyment. To achieve enjoyment through activities, usually there has to be an element of challenge or competition, with inherent potential for mastery through skill development. The concept of winning through competition or successful creative completion through mastery can enhance the individual's self-esteem.

In acute care settings, the patient can develop a bad case of passive experience. People in hospitals pay exorbitant sums to be prodded, poked and pinched by medical staff on all levels. They have their sleep disturbed by all sorts of unnatural and unfamiliar noises, and occasionally they have their worst fears confirmed. It is too easy, in any institutional setting, for a person to lose control over what is done to him or her. A person who develops weakness or disability may have even less control over how and when he or she is able to do anything. It is too easy to become passive about life in general.

Recreation can counteract this passivity. This is one area of the patient's experience where he or she can be in charge, choosing activities which permit mastery and control. Recreation can serve as an "ice-breaker," helping patients to establish rapport and thus dispelling feelings of being alone. Recreation can conjure up pleasant memories of better times. Recreation, in fact, can rekindle hope.

Activities can be adapted so that people with limiting conditions can participate. The demands of activities can be adjusted, so that persons with differing skill levels can play together. Playing pieces can be made larger or smaller, as needed. They can be weighted or altered in shape. They may be magnetized or attached to surfaces with velcro. Changes in positioning can be utilized to assist those with limited range, strength or gross mobility, to allow participation.

Occupational therapists have learned to appreciate the benefits from therapeutic recreation, and to work closely with recreation therapists in designing individual programs to help clients maximize their potential and move toward improved quality of life.

ADDITIONAL READING

Mosey, A. 1976. *Activities Therapy*. New York: Raven Press.

MacDonald, E. 1960. *Occupational Therapy in Rehabilitation*. Boston: MacMillan and Co.

Trombley, C., and Scott, A. 1979. *Occupational Therapy for Physical Dysfunction*. Baltimore, MD: William Wilkins Co.

Hopkins, H. and Smith, H. (eds.). 1983. *Occupational Therapy*. Philadelphia, PA: Lippincott and Co.

Acute Care vs. Chronic Care Models of Service to the Elderly: Implications for Therapeutic Recreation

Miriam P. Lahey

A recently published longitudinal study of predictors of success-ful aging (Vaillant and Vaillant, 1990) measures mental health sta-tus in terms of the ability to play, to work, and to love. The capacity for work (especially) and for love have long been recognized as indicators of mental health, but this study also gives prominence to the role of play. It thus focuses on a human capacity that eludes the paradigms of much health care policy and practice.

The critical role of play, of recreation and leisure, is especially integral to the physical and mental health of the elderly. For many elderly, work is a diminishing factor in self-identity and social role. The death of a spouse, the loss also of siblings and other relatives and friends, even one's changing role within the family, may mean tighter horizons to the domain of love, the complex world of per-sonal relationships, intimacy, and reciprocity. Thus, the third sphere, play, always important, becomes increasingly crucial. It also becomes, in theory at least, a sphere of greater creativity, greater self-expression and self-exploration.

In practice, however, the service model developed in acute care works against the importance of play and recreation. Moreover, this model has significant impact on chronic care of the elderly where recreation receives some degree of formal recognition, but where it

Miriam P. Lahey, PhD, is Coordinator, Recreation Program, Department of Physical Education, Recreation and Dance, Division of Professional Studies, Lehman College of CUNY, Bronx, NY, and Vice-President, Board of Directors, Women Helping Women.

is often perceived as a luxury, a time-filler, a way to manage the institutionalized elderly. Sometimes it is even considered, ironically, a kind of busy work for the elderly.

The implications of this undervaluing are particularly important to therapeutic recreation. This profession is committed to facilitating leisure experiences for variously disabled clients who need assistance in developing and/or adapting their leisure repertoire—and with that, the basic quality of their lives. When the limiting conditions of clients require clinical intervention, the function of therapeutic recreation is to help the client transcend the enveloping clinical milieu, to escape the enervating fixation on disability and on the routines of treatment.

But within the acute care model this transcending function can be reduced to a clinical outcome, a measurable product in the regimens of therapy. Thus, play becomes treatment and recreation a kind of "procedure." As a result, therapeutic recreation is brought to some hard questions about its professional purposes and identity.

These questions are not new. They are, in fact, rooted in the history of the profession, in long-standing unclarity about whether leisure is an end in itself or an instrumental means to other ends— whether "therapeutic" or "recreation" is the dominant element in the designation of the profession. Recent attention to these issues indicates that consensus is still absent (Sylvester 1987, 1989; Hemingway 1987; Lahey 1987; Reynolds and O'Morrow 1985; Halberg and Howe-Murphy 1985). Attempts to standardize professional practice through a national certification process have, in fact, only fueled the debate between those who see the therapeutic outcome as paramount and those who see outcome-driven therapy as an attempt to control or program leisure in a way that is incompatible with its very meaning.

THERAPEUTIC RECREATION: COMPETING MODELS OF THE PROFESSION

Entering the American health care system as a relatively new profession, and one without internal philosophical consensus, therapeutic recreation frequently borrows its philosophy of practice from allied fields in acute care. Since the prestige of the medical field tends to eclipse all others, the medical model is the one most frequently imitated by the therapeutic recreation profession. It is the model of preference, for example, for the National Council for Therapeutic Recreation Certification (NCTRC).

There is some irony in the fact that therapeutic recreation finds itself adapting the clinical-medical model, in the midst of increasing critique of this model. As Kass (1985) puts it, "Though it (American medicine) remains the most widely respected of professions, though it has never been more technically competent, it is in trouble, both from without and from within" (p. 157). A wide range of pressures and changes have resulted in a much more critical view of the medical establishment and its traditional authority: the patients' rights movement with its strong distrust of medical paternalism; increased scrutiny and review of physicians' decisions and practice; massive professional specialization, which fragments the caregiving relationship and turns physicians into technicians and strangers; the corporatization of medicine, which further reduces physician autonomy and creates conflicting loyalties (e.g., is one's client the patient or the HMO?); cost constraints within the system, which tie medical practice to reimbursement categories and fiscal schedules that do not automatically mirror patient need; a focus on acute care and high tech medicine that overlooks crucial areas of care and large sectors of the patient population.

On this last score, Jennings et al. (1988) point to a failure in the medical model that is sharply relevant to our discussion: "There is a specter haunting the American health care system. It is the prospect of widespread chronic illness and disability in an aging society" (p. 1).

THE CHRONIC CARE NEEDS OF THE ELDERLY

Although the Medicare program has officially singled out the health care of the elderly for special concern and, indeed, massive funding, the program is principally directed at acute care. But the health care needs of aging Americans are primarily for treatment of chronic illness. Those over 65 actually report fewer incidents of acute illness than do their younger counterparts, but, on the average, they suffer from one or more chronic illnesses, with two or more such conditions reported for those 75 and older (Jennings et al. 1988).

Among the specific chronic illnesses to which older Americans fall victim are arthritis, hearing impairment, diabetes, hypertension. All of these pathologies usually begin with slight changes in mid-life functioning, gradually increasing until there is significant impairment in the late sixties. These illnesses can be marked by such insidious onset that many initially go unreported (Adams et al. 1979). The individual affected becomes accustomed to incrementally increasing discomfort or lessening of function until the disability finally reaches severity.

Besides insidiousness and lack of clear definition at onset, chronic illness in middle and later life includes other characteristics, direct and indirect, that do not fit the categories of acute care. Directly, such illnesses are characterized by long-term duration, lack of critical medical intervention, gradual growth of debility with no promise of remission, increasing limit of function, and chronic pain. Indirectly, chronic illness brings about alterations–sometimes major–of lifestyle. The psychosocial impact of these alterations are of major concern for patients, yet they have difficulty locating appropriate help from acute care medicine. For many elderly people, the primary care setting is seen as the only health care resource, even for psychosocial problems (Kulka 1979) that they correctly identify as part of their chronic illness. Generally, however, they find that medical professionals regard such problems as outside the scope of their practice.

Because chronic illness offers no likelihood for cure, its relentless advance can stir a kind of hopelessness and helplessness. A sense of powerlessness and inevitability erodes the inner resources of the elderly, their families, other support groups, and caregivers. A mounting sense of futility, along with the incessant demands of chronic illness for attention, can create a sense that those around them do not care, that nothing will be done to bring them relief. Some elderly develop attitudes of passivity; others become more strident in their search for help and attention.

While chronic illness gives rise to psychosocial problems, these problems can create stress and precipitate further somatic complaint. On the other hand, the seriousness of underlying physiological conditions only come to be admitted by some elderly when resulting psychosocial changes erode their coping skills (Tessler and Mechanic 1978). In short, the relation of chronic illness and psychosocial disruption is complex. Many physicians are not prepared to distinguish among the different presenting problems that elderly patients bring to them. Often, psychosocial problems are treated with psychotropic medication (Hesbacher et al. 1980), which, when not carefully monitored, can have undesired side-effects, especially for older patients. At other times, the psychosocial effects of chronic illness are simply ignored when presented in the clinical setting. Borland and Jones' review of medical charts found that while 38% of patients had accompanying psychosocial problems, only 5.6% of cases were referred for treatment of such problems (1981).

ACUTE CARE VS. CHRONIC CARE
IN THE UNITED STATES

When the elderly go to primary care settings for help with the psychosocial problems of chronic illness, they are essentially responding to the structures of the health care system. In the United States, acute care settings are *the* dominant ones. The excessive, expensive, and frequently ineffective consumption of physicians' services for dealing with chronic problems is rooted in the acute care model of American medicine with its focus on the hospital and critical care.

Brown (1979) and Starr (1982) describe the historical sources of this model. In the nineteenth century, the forerunners of hospitals were religious or charitable institutions for tending the sick who had no families to care for them. Prior to the publication of Lister's work on antiseptics in 1867 and Florence Nightingale's insistence on improved hygiene, hospitals were seen as houses of rampant infection and death. A doctor might spend his entire medical career without ever going into one. Late in the last century came the adoption of aseptic techniques, the demonstration of ether as an

anesthetic, and the discovery of the X-ray. All of these developments brought about the rapid expansion in surgery and the treatment of many acute illnesses hitherto beyond the scope of medical
practice.

As hospitals gained acceptance as places for medical practice,
their admissions grew and they began, as Starr (1982) notes, "to
limit care to the more acute periods of illness . . . focusing on
curable patients rather than chronic invalids. . . . The growing
emphasis on surgery and the relief of acute illness brought about
redefinitions of purpose in hospitals" (p. 157). Essentially, hospitals began to focus on active medical and surgical treatment. Thus
the dominant pattern of modern American medicine was established: "a highly developed private sector for acute treatment and
an underdeveloped public sector for chronic care" (Starr, p. 173).

The resulting model of acute health care is characterized by
urgency, critical intervention, short-term (often life and death)
struggle. Expanding notions of social rights and employment benefits have worked, more recently, to democratize the acute care system. What once might have been seen as the privilege of a few, was
opened to most, including the rapidly increasing older population.
Finally, advances in medical technology have made it possible for
people to survive conditions previously considered fatal. These
advances have served to drive up costs, but even in the midst of
cost-containment measures, they continue to dominate health care,
creating a system that gives very low priority to chronic care needs.

Government intervention in meeting the medical needs of the
elderly has, of course, taken place within this concrete context. In
its initial form, the Social Security Act was to include health care
insurance for older Americans, but this benefit was successfully
opposed by the AMA (Mundinger 1983). Over the next 30 years
legislators continually attempted, unsuccessfully, to provide for the
health needs of older Americans, until in 1965 Medicare was passed
as Title XVIII of the Social Security Act. This was the first time the
federal government directly funded health care for a segment of the
population. In doing so, it chose to fund the existing health care
delivery system, rather than take the opportunity to reorganize the
system to meet client needs, and to make funding contingent on
updating and renewal of the system. Along with the expansion of

the medical marketplace, came a kind of guarantee of resources to hospitals. "Medicare, now in its third decade, is still virtually intact as an insurance program covering acute illness only" (Brickner et al. 1988). With the billions of dollars poured into Medicare since its inception in 1965, the pressing need of the elderly for care of chronic illness has remained largely unaddressed.

THE ADVENT OF DRGs

The runaway costs of Medicare finally led to attempts at cost containment. In 1983 the program's reimbursement system was drastically altered, from a cost-based retrospective system to a prospective payment system (PPS) introduced under Title VI of the Social Security Amendments of 1983. The new system of reimbursement is based on an average predetermined length of stay in the hospital for Medicare patients, depending on their diagnosis and their geographic location. The prospective payment system, based on diagnosis related groups (DRGs), has a number of effects on delivery of care. Since hospitals are now reimbursed on the basis of average costs of treating a person with a specific diagnosis, it has become the practice to avoid DRG-costly patients and attract DRG-profitable patients. As Smith and Reid (1984) unabashedly remark, "Clearly a strategy for maintaining financial solvency is to minimize the number of categories which offer a negative return" (p. 5).

Within the DRG system there is great pressure on doctors to keep down hospital costs. Doulenc and Dougherty (1985) cite St. Joseph Hospital in Colorado as one among others which "supplies medical staff with monthly physician-DRG profiles and has revamped salary and wage programs to tie the performance of employees to attainment of DRG goals" (p. 25). Such system-driven strategies inevitably position patients as products–costing a specific amount and yielding a calculable gain or a loss. Perhaps the most easily documented effect of DRGs is the early discharge of elderly patients. Whether they are returning to their homes or being admitted to nursing homes, patients are routinely discharged sooner than they would have been in the pre-DRG era. This is especially true of the very old, who take longer to recover from illnesses and who are more likely to be suffering from chronic conditions in addition to the acute illness for which they are admitted (Dougherty 1989). Often these patients require readmission to the hospital in a short time. As a result of premature discharge, they are frequently readmitted with a more complex diagnosis and a more profitable DRG rating.

As is usually the case, the medically indigent are particularly affected by the Prospective Payment System. Those with a history of poverty generally have poorer overall health status at hospital admission. Inevitably, they will require a longer recovery period, even though general health status on admission is not factored into the DRG system. Thus, the reimbursement system prompts hospitals to avoid such patients. In neighborhoods where the poor constitute the bulk of the population, hospitals find themselves swamped with elderly patients for whom Medicare benefits will not cover treatment costs.

DRGs: THE IMPACT ON THERAPEUTIC RECREATION

Decreased length of stay for elderly patients has increased the burden on home care and skilled nursing home services. Nursing homes are caring for more and more patients who, prior to DRGs, would still have been in hospital. Reimbursement for nursing home services is now tied to the severity of patient illness, making it more cost effective for nursing homes to serve those with acute illness rather than with chronic diseases. As a result, nursing home care is less and less available to elderly with chronic illnesses, especially those that involve cognitive functioning. Placing cognitively impaired patients is very difficult because caring for them is labor intensive, but only minimally funded by the reimbursement system.

These systematic constraints affect all health care workers. In fact, ancillary services, such as therapeutic recreation, art therapy, and occupational therapy, feel quite sharply the productivity-monitoring that comes with DRGs. As Smith and Reid (1985) note, the use of ancillary services, which have minimal return for early discharge, is directly discouraged by DRGs. For therapeutic recreation, this means pressure to demonstrate clinical outcome, in particular, contribution to quicker patient discharges. Thus the DRG system provides fiscal sanction for professionals who want to emphasize clinical results rather than the value of leisure in itself. The reimbursement mechanisms of acute care press therapeutic recreation to lay claim to direct therapeutic return, to offer measurable outcomes in the system's terms, in short, to clinicalize both its practice and its professional image. Clinicalization means, of course, that therapeutic recreation must be able to demonstrate its contribution to *medical* and *patient management* outcomes, such as early discharge. The inevitable result of this focus is deemphasis on the inherent value of leisure, whether or not it can be shown to affect such things as length of hospital stay.

One of the dangers of clinicalizing recreation services is that it can rob them of their greatest strength—the impact of true leisure and play on the lives of the elderly. Recreation is unique, especially in the clinical setting, precisely because it is not bound to specific and predictable clinical outcomes. When recreation professionals take on the role of clinicians, then, as Paul Haun (1965) suggests, they betray their gift. Patients in hospitals and residents in nursing homes are surrounded by clinicians who are busy manipulating their behavior in order to produce clinical outcomes in line with measures of "productive" treatment. Leisure offers the client one area of life that can be free from clinical manipulation, free from the "patient as product" model of service which increasingly typifies the acute care system.

The clinicalizing of recreation threatens to replace the therapeutic alliance between client and professional with a product-oriented approach (Powderly and Smith 1989). The unique relationship between client and professional in therapeutic recreation is based, in part, on personal elements (Lahey 1985). But one of these key elements, patient trust, is bound to weaken when the relationship becomes highly clinical. This is so, precisely because the DRG system defines clinical outcomes in terms of fiscally conservative care. Clinicians cannot look simply to patients' needs; they must keep a sharp eye on reimbursement categories as they respond to patients. In their turn, patients do well to observe the caveats of the marketplace in their relationship with such "suppliers" of care. If similar forces begin to shape therapeutic recreation, they will undermine the personal, free-ranging, outcome-open relationship that has characterized this particular professional-client relationship at its best.

Finally, clinicalizing recreation can lead to virtually abandoning clients who are not perceived as DRG-profitable. At a recent Mid-East Symposium on Therapeutic Recreation, a keynote speaker urging a more clinical approach insisted that it was time to realize that not everyone is a candidate for therapeutic recreation. Only those with a capacity for rehabilitation should be considered apt candidates for therapeutic intervention. But the crucial gatekeeping category, "capacity for rehabilitation," was defined in terms of measurable change in clinical status. Within the present health care system, measures of change will be tied to the highly medicalized categories and tight time limits typical of DRGs and other Medicare reimbursement formulas. In short, potential for rehabilitation is liable to be defined more by external (i.e., fiscal and medical) categories than by those indigenous to leisure and recreation. Clients who do not fit these limited categories will, like the medically indigent, be categorized out of the service system.

The great risk to the profession is that at this critical juncture in its history it will accept progressively narrow definitions of its mission. Clients who are at the "frontiers" of therapy, who need long term rehabilitative efforts, who need maintenance therapy, or who produce only small measures of progress, are liable to be seen as "outliers," as unworkable or unproductive problems for a profession driven by measurable clinical outcomes.

The chronically ill elderly are certainly prime candidates for therapeutic recreation services. Therapeutic recreation may not cure their illnesses or disabilities, but it can help improve the quality of their lives. It would be a drastic foreshortening of professional mission if the therapeutic recreation profession turned away from large numbers of the elderly because they were "beyond rehabilitation." But that is precisely the risk that the profession faces if it serves only those clients who promise "clinical outcomes" as defined within the acute-care model.

The tension between acute care and chronic care models has, therefore, deep ramifications. The mission of therapeutic recreation is to speak the value of leisure to a society that is often consumed by the calculus of outcomes, by productivity and bottom lines and cost-benefit measurements. It would signal an essential shift in mission if the profession were no longer to advocate for the elemental role of recreation in the health care of the elderly and other chronically disabled groups. If "clinical outcome" becomes the chief justification for therapeutic recreation, then the profession will no longer speak for the elusive play of leisure. Recreation will finally have locked itself into the clinical categories of the acute care system.

REFERENCES

Adams, G., Cheney C., Tustan, M., Freise, J., and Schweitzer, L. (1979). "Mental Health in Primary Care Training and Practice," *International Journal of Psychiatry in Medicine 9.*

Borland, J. and Jones, A. (1981). "Referral Patterns for Social Work Service in an Ambulatory Care Setting," *Journal of Applied Social Sciences 5.*

Brown, E. R. (1979). *Rockefeller Medicine Men: Capitalism and Medical Care in America.* Berkeley: University of California Press.

Bruckner, P., Lechich, A., Lipsman, R. and Scharer, L. (1988). *Long Term Health Care.* New York: Basic Books.

Dolenc, D. and Dougherty, C. (1985). "DRGs: The Counterrevolution in Financing Health Care," *Hastings Center Report 15.*

Dougherty, C. (1989). "Ethical Perspectives on Prospective Payment," *Hastings Center Report 19.*

Halberg, K. and Howe-Murphy, R. (1985). "The Dilemma of an Unresolved Philosophy in Therapeutic Recreation," *Therapeutic Recreation Journal 19.*

Haun, P. (1965). *Recreation: A Medical Viewpoint.* New York: Teachers College Press.

Hemingway, J. (1987). "Building a Philosophical Defense of Therapeutic Recreation: The Case of Distributive Justice," in C. Sylvester (ed.) *Philosophy of Therapeutic Recreation: Ideas and Issues.* Alexandria, VA: National Therapeutic Recreation Society/National Recreation and Parks Association.

Hesbacher, P., Rickels, K., Morris, R., Newman, H., Rosenfeld, H. (1986). "Psychiatric Illness in Family Practice," *Journal of Clinical Psychiatry 4.*

Jennings, B., Callahan, D., and Caplan, A. L. (1988). "Ethical Challenges of Chronic Illness," *Hastings Center Report 20.*

Kass, L. R. (1985). *Toward a More Natural Science.* New York: The Free Press.

Kulka, R., Veroff, J., and Douvan, E. (1979). "Social Class and the Use of Professional Help for Personal Problems," *Journal of Health and Social Behavior 20.*

Lahey, M. P. (1987). "The Ethics of Intervention in Therapeutic Recreation," in

C. Sylvester (ed.) *Philosophy of Therapeutic Recreation: Ideas and Issues.* Alexandria, VA: National Therapeutic Recreation Society/National Recreation and Parks Association.

Mundinger, M. (1983). *Home Care Controversy.* Rockville, MD: Aspen.

Powderly, K. E. and Smith, E. (1989). "The Impact of DRGs on Health Care Workers and Their Clients," *Hastings Center Report* 19.

Reynolds, R. P. and O'Morrow, G. S. (1985). *Problems, Issues and Concepts in Therapeutic Recreation.* Englewood Cliffs, NJ: Prentice Hall.

Starr, P. (1982). *The Social Transformation of American Medicine.* New York: Basic Books.

Smith, H. and Reid, R. (1984). "Short and Long Run Management Strategies for DRGs," *Hospital Topics.*

Sylvester, C. (1987). "Therapeutic Recreation and the End of Leisure," in C. Sylvester (ed.) *Philosophy of Therapeutic Recreation: Ideas and Issues.* Alexandria, VA: National Therapeutic Recreation Society/National Recreation and Parks Association.

Sylvester, C. (1989). "Impressions of the Intellectual Past and Future of Therapeutic Recreation: Implications for Professionalization," in D. M. Compton (ed.) *Issues in Therapeutic Recreation: A Profession in Transition.*

Tessler, R. and Mechanic, D. (1978). "Psychological Distress and Perceived Health Status," *Journal of Health and Social Behavior* 19.

Vaillant, C. E. and Vaillant, C. O. (1990), "Natural History of Male Psychological Health, XII: A 45-year Study of Predictors of Successful Aging at Age 65," *American Journal of Psychiatry* 47.

Surviving a Fate Worse than Death: The Plight of the Homebound Elderly

Stuart Waldman

For the elderly person who can no longer survive independently in the community, being confined to home may be a necessity. For confused and disoriented persons, attempting to make sense of the incomprehensible, the need to be confined to home may be an even less understandable experience. Where once these populations may have been hospitalized or institutionalized for indefinite periods of time, new methods of cost analysis and funding have meant the reemergence of community care (Goldstein 1987). More specifically, the hospital system's Diagnostic Resource Groups assign a specific level of reimbursement for particular diagnostic categories. The longer a patient is in the hospital, the higher the cost; therefore, early discharge means greater profits for the hospital (Shumer 1988). Nursing homes, reimbursed in New York State through a system of Resource Utilization Groups, receive funding on the documented need of care for each of their residents. While this system sounds logical, it may facilitate rejection of potential clients by nursing homes on the basis of lower reimbursement level (Kaufman 1988). Thus, both the prematurely discharged hospital patient and the prospective nursing home resident may find themselves at home.

Home care programs and agencies have developed in order to meet the diverse health care needs of this "at-home" population. These agencies provide visiting nurses, social workers, rehabilitation specialists, and homemaker services and arrange for medical

Stuart Waldman, MS, is Director of Activities, Menorah Home and Hospital, Brooklyn, NY.

appointments. These services may be funded through private payment, through insurance, or through Medicaid (Shumer 1989).

Confined to their homes, perhaps living alone, and often unable to experience their customary and familiar community-related routines, these elderly persons may suffer a profound sense of grief, a loss of social being. Many behaviors observed within the homebound population are remarkably similar to those observed by Kübler-Ross (1969) among the dying. Is the prognosis, therefore, a social death? Can the homebound patient survive physical illness and succumb to social death?

In order to understand this social phenomenon, it is necessary to further examine the psychological and emotional experiences of a population so different that they cannot, on their own, leave their homes, yet who are not ill enough to be institutionalized where socialization could be fostered, facilitated and encouraged. Claiming that denial is often the first stage in the response of the dying to their approaching death, Kübler-Ross (1969) believes that the denial of the illness and prognosis is often coupled with isolation. By isolating oneself, reminders of one's condition and fate are made to vanish. Often the initial response of the homebound person is similar to this. Attempts by friends and family members to visit, according to Shumer (1989), are rejected with excuses such as "not feeling up to it," or "when I'm better." Even those home health care personnel assigned to a case are shunned. Isolation, truly a social, or rather, antisocial response, develops, despite attempts by caregivers to reach out to the client.

Anger, which Kübler-Ross (1969) describes as the second stage of response to dying, is often manifested in such questions as "how can this happen to me?" Home health care workers report that they have been verbally abused by their clients. Occasionally visiting nurses are hit, scratched, and attacked; family members are blamed (Shumer 1989). This antisocial behavior may further promote isolation.

Kübler-Ross (1969) sees a third stage when the anger begins to subside–bargaining. Most often unrealistic, a specific one-time bargain is proposed in which good behavior (in one or many areas) is promised in exchange for good health: "If I get better, I'll never be nasty again," or, perhaps, "If I do my therapy, I'll get better, and I'll never . . ." Thus, the antisocial behavior may seem to subside. Caution is needed in making such an observation. The patient may allow social interaction for the purpose of the bargain. A therapist or nurse may visit, but apart from these specified caregivers, social isolation is maintained.

Isolation and withdrawal continue through the next stage, which Kübler-Ross (1969) sees as depression. For the ailing homebound patient who may be experiencing this stage because of a diagnosis of physical illness, the loss of the social presence can only exacerbate his or her depression. Confinement, and the inability to function in a familiar social environment may, in fact, contribute to even greater depression. Manifestations of depression may result in even further social withdrawal, further withdrawal from meaningful leisure activity, extreme loss of appetite, and a general lack of desire to thrive.

Some homebound persons do survive these stages, and, according to Kübler-Ross (1969), accept their condition and their fate. So, too, on a social level some come to accept confinement, learn how to facilitate leisure and social experience, manipulate systems to engage special escorts and transportation out of their confinement (Shumer 1989).

What about those who do not seem to reach the stage of acceptance? As leisure service professionals, how do we address these stages when they are related to a purely medical condition? By the mere definition of leisure as an activity, a period of discretionary time, or an experience that requires freedom of choice and intrinsic satisfaction (Kelly 1982), we have already offered the possibility of an intervention that can become therapeutic. Those involved in a therapeutic milieu direct their efforts toward the leisurability model, including therapy affecting functional behavior, leisure education, and the facilitation of voluntary recreation participation. The community recreation specialist focuses attention on the provision of a variety of opportunities. What the institutional and community leisure specialist have in common is the facilitation of leisure experience.

The leisure service professional can play an important part in responding to the client's movement through the stages described by Kübler-Ross (1969). The isolation of the denial stage can be addressed by gradually building and developing a trusting relationship, by offering moral support, by providing leisure counseling. The leisure professional may further explore attitudes and possibilities, may promote skill acquisition, and eventually provide opportunities for social involvement and interaction. These opportunities may engage others with similar medical conditions, thereby not only facilitating a leisure experience, but also building peer group support.

How do we address anger that may be manifested in verbal or other behaviors? Often by creating an atmosphere where it can be expressed; by focusing energies where anger can be released in a more constructive manner–wedging clay, hitting a punching bag, or engaging in appropriate exercise routines.

Depression may be expressed through unrealistic guilt or shame for past deeds, perhaps even leisure and recreational experiences (sexual habits, cheating at games, over-exertion). The reality of lost opportunities or the emotional anticipation of future losses plays a major role. Again, the provision of opportunities, either through adaptation of old skills or the teaching of new skills can build a leisure repertoire in which the client can have a sense of a new chance.

In brief, then, leisure services offer a variety of opportunities–to take risks, to experience excitement, to gain mastery. All these opportunities emphasize the freedom to be responsible for and have control over one's own destiny. Joy and pleasure follow, with a resulting increase of relaxation, reduction of stress, and, finally, building of an affirmative attitude.

These positive aspects are active concerns of the leisure service provider whose goal is to contribute to the client's quality of life. For many "special populations" there are leisure professionals who have become familiar with all the needs of the client group and so are able to design appropriate interventions. Some of the "emerging special populations," however, may be neglected by the profession, falling between the cracks of service delivery, as it were. Those whom the hospital discharges (perhaps prematurely), whom nursing homes refuse and rehabilitation centers reject, those who must remain at home–such clients are not part of the traditional health care treatment pattern, and thus may be neglected by the health care team, including the recreation professionals. Some are wise in the ways of leisure, and over the years have developed leisure repertoires upon which they can rely. But for those who are grieving over their medical condition and what may indeed be a social death, leisure death may be inevitable.

Home health care programs address many needs of the home-bound population, some of which are reimbursed by insurance. Generally, however, leisure needs are not covered. Such programs seem to perceive the client only in terms of the medical diagnosis, rather than as a whole human being. Adult day care programs address all the human needs of their clients (Goldstein 1987). But these programs are few in comparison to the great need for community care. Shumer (1989) finds that members of her home health care team are concerned about their clients' social isolation, unconstructive use of time, depression, and extreme anger. All team members felt that a leisure specialist would be a welcome addition to the team. But who will pay?

What can the leisure specialist do? Those involved with community recreation can further explore ideas and ways of addressing the needs of these members of the community who are daily increasing in number. Those involved in therapeutic recreation can explore avenues in facilities and organizations that can be expanded to accommodate a population for whom leisure and recreation are an urgent necessity. For those who perceive leisure and recreation as an important aspect of life, and the right of all people, advocacy is essential. On a final note, there are some who feel that being institutionalized in a hospital or nursing home may be a fate worse than death–that may be an anticipatory perception. Many claim that they would feel happier in their own homes. Often these are responses of people who have not experienced the isolation, the death of social existence, the loss of leisure and recreation which can come to the homebound.

REFERENCES

Goldstein, R. 1987. Interview with Rose Goldstein, Director of Social Services, Jewish Home and Hospital for Aged, Bronx, New York.

Kaufman, S. 1988. Interview with Sandra Kaufman, Director of Admissions, Kingsbridge Heights Nursing Home, Bronx, New York.

Kelly, J. R. 1982. *Leisure.* Englewood Cliffs, NJ: Prentice-Hall.

Kübler-Ross, E. 1969. *On Death and Dying.* New York: Macmillan.

Shumer, A. 1989. Interview with Arlene Shumer, Director of the Long-Term Home Health Care Program, Kingsbridge Heights Nursing Home, Bronx, New York.

Therapeutic Group Activities
with Alzheimer's Patients

Sidney R. Saul

The helping professions always seek out the residual health and strengths of an individual when attempting to cope with any presenting condition or illness. This is true for the patient and family suffering from Alzheimer's disease, as it is for any others. Because the nature of the disease is so devastating and the disease itself incurable, a diagnosis of Alzheimer's disease usually leads the family and the patient to believe that there is no help and that little, if anything, can be done. Helping efforts are usually focused on the family and/or the caring person. The patient is given up for lost.

Although at present the disease itself is indeed incurable, there are many things that can be done to alleviate the distress and suffering of the patient, as well as of the family. Therefore, intervention is valid, and it is incumbent upon health professionals to learn about and improve the victim's life circumstances.

A few brief words about the disease are in order here. Alzheimer's disease is a neurological condition that affects specific neurotransmitters in the brain. Envision an old-time telephone switchboard where the operator plugs in jacks to connect lines of communication. Similarly, the brain sends messages to the rest of the body via neurotransmitters. Imagine the telephone jacks beginning to rust and the messages coming through with decreasing clarity, until the rust becomes so thick that no contact is made at all. This gives us a picture of how plaques and tangles around the nerve endings of the brain gradually cause confusion and disorientation in

Sidney R. Saul, EdD, is affiliated with Kingsbridge Heights Nursing Home, Bronx, NY.

the patient. The process continues until all memory is lost. Body functions begin to slow down, and eventually the person dies.

The disease is initially insidious and silent and usually not recognized until it is fairly well along. It continues to progress gradually but relentlessly until death, the whole process lasting anywhere from one to fifteen years. Hence the appellation, "The Silent Epidemic." Diagnosis is extremely difficult. It is often made through the process of excluding all other possibilities. Definitive diagnosis can only be made upon biopsy of the brain at autopsy.

There is no cure. There is no medication to halt or even to alter the process. The diagnosis is often an educated guess. Care must be taken to ensure that the diagnosis is not made hastily or erroneously. As if this were not enough, Alzheimer's disease may be accompanied by a range of physical and emotional conditions, which complicate the patient's total condition and affect behavior. These accompanying conditions, when identified, may be treatable, thus alleviating at least part of the problem (e.g., drug interactions, depression, malnutrition, and a variety of physical illnesses).

Caregivers need to be aware of, and take into account the impact of this massive and emotional blow upon the family homeostasis. If possible, the worker should encourage and help plan for relief of the relentless caregiving the family must supply. The patient is also affected by the additional tensions in the home and can be helped by help given the family.

The "treatment" of the Alzheimer's patient and the family must, by necessity, be an interdisciplinary effort appropriately involving neurology, internal medicine, psychiatry, nursing, nutrition, social work, the rehabilitation therapies, and, significantly, therapeutic recreation.

At the Maimonides Community Mental Health Center in Brooklyn, we created an outpatient treatment program for 15 confused and disoriented people, most of whom had been diagnosed as having Alzheimer's disease. All were living at home. It is believed that there are more Alzheimer's patients living at home than are living in institutions.

This program was conducted for three hours per day. In addition, it involved about one hour of transportation each way, thus comprising a five-hour day. This was just about as much as the patient could accept. The program, therefore, provided a daily five-hour respite for the patient who was taken out of the tense climate at home and given an opportunity to relax. The family was required to provide one day a week of volunteer assistance to the group. It was stipulated that this volunteer would be assigned to work with a patient other than the family member. This assured adequate "hands-on" coverage for the program, while providing an opportunity to teach the caring persons some skills that could be used in helping the patient at home.

The day was structured for a range of therapeutic modalities and interventions. Both patients and staff worked intensely during the three contact hours of the program. A caring person rode in the program's bus both morning and afternoon, thus providing staff contact during the entire five hours each day.

The patients arrived at 10 a.m. The first hour was spent in getting reacquainted. This was a daily activity as these patients would forget each other within minutes after leaving the bus in the afternoon. Group therapy, geared to whatever topics the patients were capable of discussing, was usually conducted in the morning. Since there were clearly two levels of functioning, two therapy groups were created and met in two separate rooms. Content of the therapy group session was developed out of immediate and presenting situations whenever possible. Open communication with families, as well as staff awareness of ongoing relationships, contributed to staff sensitivity to problems, incidents, and needs.

From 11 a.m. until noon, the entire group went to lunch. Although the staff, the kitchen staff included, had been prepared to serve and even to feed the group members (if necessary), the patients rose to the occasion from the very first day. They went on line, cafeteria style, and, with staff supervision, chose their own food, carried their trays to the tables, selected their own tablemates, and ate, unaided. Finally, they bussed their own tables. Mealtime became an important part of their social, as well as nutritional, therapy. It also provided an opportunity to do something for themselves, something not often practiced at home.

After lunch, the group participated in planned, therapeutic activities. Although these activities were adapted to the cognitive level of the group, they were conducted on an adult level, without infantilizing the participants. What was needed was for the staff to be creative in adapting activities, so that a variety of possibilities was discovered.

For stimulating memory, the staff developed cognitive activities such as a "memory wall" (pictures and slogans of earlier times, drawn from discussions with the patients); the use of alphabet letters to create words and names; reading exercises; writing, counting and short-term memory games.

For strengthening the sense of identity and earlier roles, the staff used full-length and hand mirrors, grooming activities, discussions about former experiences of the patients, celebrations of birthdays and holidays, pictures of self and family.

For confirming the patient's sense of self through roles and tasks in the present, the staff helped each person choose a "job" related, when possible, to an earlier, familiar role or task. This became a daily responsibility for each patient; e.g., sorting magazines, distributing name-tags, watering plants, feeding fish.

In all activities, efforts were directed toward maximizing present memory so that the patients experienced the joys of the moment. Existing social skills were employed and strengthened through dance therapy, social dancing, discussions, group dining, and parties.

Physical exercise sessions, so very important for this group, were conducted every day. Balloons were used, as were very light beach balls. Games evolved around such equipment, involving the patients in social as well as physical interchange. These activities provoked fun and laughter and feelings of camaraderie, all of which had been lost to some degree as part of the process of their illness. Crafts, mural-painting, and games contributed to the patients' feelings of constructiveness and creativeness.

These and countless other activities that caring and innovative recreation therapists know how to develop are the tools through which the goals of treatment can be reached and measured. Not only do these activities strengthen the patient's sense of self and offer opportunities for socialization and "normal" life experiences, they also help to alleviate anxiety and depression, and contribute to control of behavior and impulse.

The attitude of staff is crucially important in such a program. The concern, approval, acceptance, interest, and affection of staff, reflected from member to member and within the group as a whole, are critical therapeutic elements.

The following letter, written by the daughter of one of the patients, describes the impact of the program on the patient as well as the family.

Dear Dr. Saul:

I would like to share some thoughts and observations with you as to the progress of my mother, a patient in your group for six months now. When you interviewed my mother at the end of March, you expressed your belief that her illness was advanced, and that I should expect no cures or miracles. I agreed with your diagnosis because I have lived with her almost seven years now and I am her sole care person. I have watched her decline to the point where she no longer recognized me and every room in the house became strange to her. She was unresponsive, closed-up, something very close to a zombie. It's as if she were in a coma with her eyes open.

She started in your group in May and the change in her is nothing short of miraculous. She has become a social butterfly, responsive, eager to participate, helpful to other patients, and a changed person at home. When I speak to her, she becomes alert and answers me!

Her very first day in your group was a milestone in our house. She came home and said nothing, but that night at dinner (almost six hours after she came home) she said, "we had so much fun today—all we did was laugh. I played ball and had a good time. I even danced." This was the first sentence she completed in more than a year and it was about something that happened hours earlier. My teen-age son and I were amazed. Neighbors notice how sociable she is now—she waves and smiles and says she is fine when asked.

In my opinion, had she never been exposed to your group, she would have shrivelled and declined so severely by now that she would probably be bedridden. Your group is keeping her alive physically, mentally, and psychologically. She is thriving on it. It is vital that she be there every day and I schedule all her appointments so we will not miss a session.

To be perfectly honest with you, I originally thought of this group as a blessing for me–a relief from the 36-hour day–but after observing her change, I realize that it is way beyond that, and how vital it is to her well-being.

Well, so many words to say simply–bless you, bless your loving and caring staff, and bless the work you are doing.

Sincerely——

Can there possibly be a better, more positive evaluation for the program than such a letter, which expresses the feelings of so many of our patients' families?

Meaningful Life Activities
for Elderly Residents
of Residential Health Care Facilities

Shura Saul

Please consider, for a moment, your personal answer to this question. "What makes life meaningful to you?" Undoubtedly, everyone's answer will be different in the specifics, but in general, all will probably conform somehow to Maslow's hierarchical listing of common human needs (Maslow 1954). Somewhere in the meaning of your life will be such items as physical health, safety and security, affectionate and loving relationships, components of self- and social esteem, and finally, those particular dimensions of your own personality—your own interests, your own dreams, hopes and expectations for pinnacle self-actualization, to be all you want to be, all you can be!

Now, please try a second question. Consider that your circumstances have changed. You no longer live in your own home, but rather in a strange place, a small room you share with someone you don't know very well. Your body no longer serves you as well. You depend on other people not very familiar to you for the most elemental and fundamental activities of your life. Someone helps you bathe, dress, eat, perhaps even walk. Someone cooks for you and decides on your menu. Someone else cleans your room, cares for your clothing, perhaps even tells you what to wear. And finally the rhythm of your days and nights is no longer yours to orchestrate. You conform to a generalized, communal situation in which your dependency is the single most determining factor of your moment-to-moment existence.

Shura Saul, DSW, is Consultant, Kingsbridge Heights Nursing Home, Bronx, NY.

Think about that. Now, what makes life meaningful to you?

This second question is asked, because in discussing activities for residents, people must be understood in terms of their individual and group needs at this particular point in their life development.

Aging is, by now, accepted as a process of human existence. Being old is viewed as a stage of human development that presents the individual with certain gains, losses, and challenges for adaptation and growth. Being old and a resident of an institution becomes a particular challenge in the aging of some elderly people who must shape their responses within the framework of their own life circumstances, past and present. These are the last years of their lives. The severe losses they have already experienced are prelude to their final loss, that is, loss of life itself. Because aging is so truly an individual process, each person will have individual and different responses to the challenge of living in a health care facility.

None of us can answer the second question accurately, for at this point in our own development, the circumstances can only be imagined despite our familiarity with experiences of others. However, having accepted responsibility for helping residents, we must try to begin where they are, so that our ideas and our work become relevant and acceptable.

People come to live in a health care facility because their primary need is for health care. This fact has been forced upon them and their needs recognized to the point where they have relinquished much control over other aspects of their lives in order to survive. Survival, you see, is the base line of the Maslow hierarchy!

Yet, survival is not enough. Total health depends upon a meaningful existence. Enter then, the workers who offer meaningful activity to the residents. So far, the use of the term recreation has been avoided, and for a specific reason. "Recreation" is defined by Webster as "refreshment in mind or body, as after work, by some form of play, amusement or relaxation. . . . as games, sports, hobbies, reading, walking." Synonyms offered by Webster are amusement, diversion, entertainment, pastime, sport (Webster 1983).

Certainly, many activities in health care facilities are definable under these headings. However, it is posited here that the responsibility of activities workers is far more complex and extensive than diversion, play, or amusement. All disciplines in the facility are charged with the task of replacing some of the losses suffered by the residents. Rehabilitation specialists emphasize the importance of maximizing a person's strengths and abilities in order to achieve the highest possible level of independent functioning. Health care workers are encouraged to offer opportunities for residents to make choices, even seemingly simple ones, e.g., in clothing and food.

Recreation therapists do more than "refresh or amuse" the residents. They help to replace some lost opportunities for purposeful living. A range of such available activities becomes a significant component of the unified effort to create a totally healthy living situation. Ways must be found to serve all the residents through a diversified program for groups and for individuals.

The extent of this challenge is enormous and exhilarating to the creative worker. The range of possibilities is limited only by the human imagination which is just about limitless.

Let's identify a few significant goals and related activities. Although not always easy, the following illustrative examples have all been implemented.

A primary goal concerns the loss of control over life, experienced by most residents. Certain controls can be restored through selected activities. On an individual level, therapeutic recreation professionals explore a person's interests, and plan, together with the resident, to fulfill these. This also restores a person's individuality and sense of self, another important program goal. On the group level, wherever possible, activities should be planned with the residents, who should be involved in implementing and evaluating the programs. This approach offers residents active control.

A Resident Council can become a most imaginative channel for group planning. The council must be viewed by the facility and the staff as a vehicle for resident expression–expression, not only in the form of complaints (and they are important), but also through a broad range of activities, both within and beyond the institution. Some exciting events are illustrative.

The Coalition of Institutionalized Aged and Disabled works with resident groups to lobby for relevant legislation, or with residents who have been successful in such efforts on their own behalf. Residents have participated in workshops and Senior Speak-Outs at conferences of community groups such as the Bronx-North Manhattan Coalition for the Elderly and Long-Term Care.

Along similar lines, a number of residents from the Kingsbridge Heights Health Care Facilities attended the annual CIAD citywide conference on the Resident Bill of Rights. They then organized a meeting within their own facility at which they reported on this conference to other residents and to staff. Follow-up activities included "rap sessions" between staff and residents and discussions about inservice training. These activities brought staff and residents to a new closeness and understanding. They also gave the residents an opportunity to participate significantly with others in their world.

Another example: in an effort to improve resident behavior in the elevators, a Resident Education Committee developed a skit on this theme and performed it with great success at a series of resident community meetings. This is an instance where a small group activity was important to the entire facility. The elevator problem was not solved for all time, but indeed, there was some improvement. This Committee continued to meet and make recommendations for changed behavior of residents and staff, e.g., for the latter to be more quiet during the shift changes, and for oiling of squeaky wheels on carts brought to the units during quiet hours. These are some of the ways residents can take responsibility in the communal living situation.

On an individual level, Mr. G., a blind resident, complained that his life was now worthless. It was suggested that he could do what he had always done as a fervent activist, namely, make a contribution to his fellow residents because of his intellectual ability and experience. He agreed to become the editor of the resident newspaper. His editorials were read with interest by residents and staff.

Such activities are directed toward restoring feelings of self-esteem, developing roles and status within the facility, establishing a sense of control in one's life, and developing a true sense of belonging in one's own home.

To be valid and successful, such activities depend upon several preexisting factors. The first requirement is the sincerity of the institution in fostering such programs and the sincerity of the staff toward them. Another requirement is the belief by the staff and administration that residents have the right, the strength, and the capacity to function on their own behalf.

Sometimes it may seem easier to infantilize frail, old, dependent people than to encourage their functioning as autonomous adults. Yet, they are adults, and caring workers must avoid the reinforcement of learned helplessness that often accompanies dependency.

Strengthening memory and intellect, encouraging their use, showing each resident that he or she is still capable of thought and expression are other important processes. Examples have already been given for mentally alert residents, but the goal applies equally to the confused and disoriented. As in physical rehabilitation, it becomes a matter of gearing expectations realistically to the individuals (Saul 1987a).

Even confused residents can be encouraged to think and operate somehow on their own behalf. For example, a new administrator was introduced to a group of residents meeting in their weekly group discussion session. The leader introduced him and asked the group what they would like to say. One confused woman said, "I'd like to suggest that you be kind and gentle with us, and that when you teach the staff, teach them to find the best in each person." There was a round of applause from the other residents.

Kingsbridge Heights Health Care Facilities has produced a series of videotapes entitled "We'll Help You Think." These tapes demonstrate ways in which a group of deeply confused and disoriented residents can be encouraged to exercise their cognitive abilities (Kingsbridge Heights 1983).

The taped sessions involve residents in such exercises as group problem solving, reminiscence, identifying common objects, associative memory exercises, and social interchange. While there may be minimum carryover, there is a strong sense of achievement in the process, an important improvement in self-esteem, and a significant emotional afterglow–all valid goals for a recreation program.

Another goal is to help restore residents' sense of individuality. The person may be helped to rediscover him or herself through continuity of interest, of capacity, of uniqueness. One example is the case mentioned earlier, Mr. G., the editor. Another is Mrs. N., who was a high-functioning person with an interesting past in the entertainment world in Europe. She joined a poetry group, and soon began writing beautiful poetry. She told us that she'd been a writer in her own language, but until this point, many years after coming to this country, she had never expected to be able to compose in English. The poetry group had given her a new, strengthened sense of herself and her creative talents.

Like the other goals, this one is not limited to high-functioning residents. Working with a group of mentally frail old women in the Royal Edinburgh Hospital in Scotland, I introduced myself by writing my name on a large piece of oaktag and then asked the patients whether they would like to write their names as well. Each of these confused women agreed, and proudly did so. Individuality was reinforced, as was each women's sense of self. Their nurses were amazed. They hadn't known their patients were capable of writing their names.

The arts, an integral component of our humanness and a universal means of communication, can serve as a vehicle toward this goal. Sound, vision, touch, movement, all these activities become media through which people express their thoughts, their insights, and especially their feelings (Saul 1987).

Music, movement, and the graphic arts circumvent traditional verbal communication. Poetry and drama diversify, transcend, and extend traditional use of words. Feelings are communicated with great power and there are endless possibilities for self-expression, insights, and meaningful learning. However, there must be a truly creative approach to the art forms. The full dignity and power of the medium must be authentically utilized on an adult level. Then the results are beautiful artistic products, but even more importantly, bring meaning to the lives of the individuals.

Resident art work may be framed and displayed throughout the facility. One resident, whose reputation was not the happiest, joined the art program. Although she had never painted before, she was clearly quite talented. She gave gifts of her paintings to residents and staff. Needless to say, her status, as well as her self-image, was much improved.

A group of depressed women participated in a poetry group, developed a poem about growing old, and performed it for the other residents. The performance was videotaped and the entire staff had the opportunity to view it. Again, the self- and social esteem of these people rose markedly.

A dramatics group was developed by a talented staff member, and the residents produced an abbreviated version of a Broadway musical for resident and staff enjoyment. A fine use of dramatics is improvisation, which permits various situations to be played out, and helps people to feel better about themselves (Stern 1987).

Educational activities are important. Colleges have brought their classrooms and teachers into the facility. The residents enjoyed their learning experiences and contact with the college. A course in drama literature was conducted for an integrated group of blind and sighted residents. It began with a study of "Oedipus Rex" and ended with the plays of Arthur Miller. The course was attended by a very diverse group of residents, some with college backgrounds, some without. To this day, residents recall the course with pleasure.

Intergenerational experiences are exciting. Young people and children of all ages participate in many ways. Nursery age children are "adopted" as grandchildren, and residents become "foster grandparents." The visits between these age groups are delightful and beneficial to all.

There can be more profound dimensions in such experiences. Some residents can develop helping roles such as tutoring youngsters who need special help with school work. Others develop encouraging relationships with needy young people. One resident at Kingsbridge Heights tutored several staff members working toward their high school equivalency. An oral history program brought City College students to learn about older peoples' experiences of earlier times. The Bronx High School of Science sent a study group to learn about immigration. The students put out a pamphlet on the subject, and both generations derived profit from the sharing. The residents gained self-esteem and a sense of purpose. The students developed new perspectives.

Many, many more such examples can be cited, despite the fact that most recreation departments are understaffed, underfunded, and at times underappreciated. Recreation professionals face the many challenges of bringing meaning to the lives of nursing home residents. They are a vital part of the multidisciplinary team endeavoring to bring new life to the years spent in an institutional setting. Their task is to enable residents to find meaning, refreshment in mind or body, as Webster puts it, and the freedom and joy which are the hallmarks of leisure.

REFERENCES

Kingsbridge Heights Health Care Facilities. 1983. *We'll Help You Think.* Video-taped series, produced with Lehman College, Audio-Visual Department.

Maslow, A. 1954. *Motivation and Personality.* Princeton, NJ: Van Nostrand.

Saul, S. 1987. "The Arts as Therapeutic Modalities." In B. MacLennon, S. Saul, and M. Weiner, (eds.), *Group Therapies for the Elderly.* Hartford, CT: International Universities Press.

Saul, S. R. 1987a. "Group Therapy with Confused and Disoriented Elderly." In B. MacLennon, S. Saul, and M. Weiner, (eds.), *Group Therapies for the Elderly.* Hartford, CT: International Universities Press.

Stern, R. 1987. "Drama Gerontology: Group Therapy Through Counseling and Drama Techniques." In B. MacLennon, S. Saul, and M. Weiner, (eds.), *Group Therapies for the Elderly.* Hartford, CT: International Universities Press.

Webster, N. 1983. *Webster's New Universal Unabridged Dictionary.* Second Edition. New York: Simon & Schuster.

From Custodial Care to Quality Care: Implications for the Therapeutic Recreation Professional

Fred S. Greenblatt

"Recreation" and its implications have probably existed as far back as the beginning of civilization. However, the ability to define clearly what we mean by "recreation" did not exist until much later (Greenblatt 1988).

The use of activities varied among civilizations and cultures. Songs and costumes were used by primitive peoples to ward off demons and evil spirits.

Later, in America, industrialization fostered greater needs for personal, physical, and psychological satisfaction, which, in turn, resulted in a new meaning for "recreation." Recreation was being accepted as an avenue for achieving satisfaction and enjoyment.

As America matured, so did its concern for the welfare of its citizens. Hospitals provided recreation services to wounded military and began hiring hospital recreation workers.

Concern for the mentally retarded expanded as well. "The public began to realize that a well-organized recreation program could accomplish much in the way of a better lifestyle for all Americans" (Greenblatt 1988).

Societal changes continued to foster significant developments in the therapeutic recreation profession. The recognition of therapeutic recreation as an intervention that contributed to the promotion of health and prevention of further illness or disability led to an expansion of services into community areas and city agencies as well as hospital settings.

Fred S. Greenblatt, MS, CTRS, is Director of Activities, The Jewish Home and Hospital for Aged, Bronx, NY.

By the 1960s, the National Therapeutic Recreation Society (NTRS) was established to help satisfy the needs and interests of recreation professionals involved in recreation in a variety of human service areas. Since that time, a variety of issues and beliefs have been debated based upon the goals and objectives of the therapeutic recreation profession. Some believed recreation could be seen as a "therapy" by itself, while others believed therapeutic effects were the precipitating factors that promoted good health and a better psychological state.

The diversity of these debates resulted in certain underlying basic principles upon which our current ideologies rest. These include the beliefs by many that (1) recreation is a specific and systematic process through which its therapeutic intervention helps create certain behavioral changes in the client; (2) therapeutic recreation cannot be considered "curative" in itself; (3) therapeutic recreation as a "therapeutic intervention" helps create a milieu necessary to facilitating positive behavioral changes of the recreation client; (4) recreation therapists work with remaining abilities and skills unaffected by disease or illness; and (5) working with the positive aspects of one's personality and physical strength helps facilitate the growth and development of the "total being or individual" (Greenblatt 1988).

These issues and beliefs, which culminated in a philosophical statement of the National Therapeutic Recreation Society, have greatly affected the delivery of therapeutic recreation services.

While our beliefs and philosophies were diversified, our concern for quality care was always a common thread. Whether recreation was viewed as a "therapy" itself or whether it was seen as a precipitating factor for positive change, improving quality of life (especially for those with limitations) remained a central focus or goal.

By the 1970s, societal changes precipitated yet another concern that had great implications for the recreation profession. By this time, there was an increased need to control the spiraling costs of health care now provided to all Americans living both in the community or within the walls of an institutional or hospital setting. Measures were taken to control the cost of health care, hopefully without having a negative impact on the quality of care or the quality of life of individuals with disabilities. Quality assurance, which has been in existence for many years, began to emerge as an important concern (Riley 1987).

The continued advent of cost control through state and federal regulations has had a tremendous impact upon society, especially for those elderly living in long-term care facilities or nursing homes. New government reimbursement systems (i.e., RUGS) have created additional changes for long-term care facilities, which are now forced to admit only the sickest patients. These trends continue to affect the delivery of therapeutic recreation services within the long-term care facility. Both the increased cost of health care and the need to service an even sicker nursing home population presents a greater challenge to the recreation professional.

Between the unparalleled changes and the concern for reimbursement dollars, the humanistic care of the institutionalized frail elderly is greatly affected. Now, more than ever before, we are caught between the need to care for the sicker elderly and the ability to provide high level quality care and recreation programming through a tightly scrutinized cost containment system.

Thus, new government reimbursement systems and the admission of sicker residents to nursing homes have contributed to the changing role of the long-term care facility and its impact on therapeutic recreation. The institution, whose original responsibility was to provide basic shelter and custodial care, has now become a multilevel agency providing health services, adult day care, and home health care, among other services. "Old folks homes" have begun to emerge from this experience as new "geriatric centers," and have, in the process, drastically modified their traditional pseudofamilial atmosphere to one more closely resembling a treatment milieu (Hammerman 1974). These changes are providing the impetus to redefine quality care through the delivery of therapeutic recreation services.

WHAT IS QUALITY CARE?

As stated earlier, although recreation has probably existed for thousands of years, it was not clearly defined until much later. The same probably holds true for our role in caring for the elderly.

Although we have always provided some kind of "care" to the elderly (whether it be custodial or treatment oriented), it is difficult to define exactly what we mean by "quality of care." Addressing the same question more directly, to what degree does the therapeutic recreation profession assure quality service to its clientele? As Riley (1987) and others point out, the response of recreation professionals is often that, although they "feel" they provide quality oriented services, they cannot substantiate this belief with a great deal of evidence.

Although quality has certain characteristics, such as excellence or goodness, its meaning as a service varies among health care professionals. Quality care to the recreation professional might include the opportunity for achievement of success in a recreation activity that helps the impaired person strengthen and use remaining abilities, providing an increased feeling of self-sufficiency. On the other hand, the business person might view quality as achieving a zero deficit and high morale of staff.

Donabedian (1978) sees quality of care as encompassing certain elements. The technical or scientific element addresses the balance between risks and benefits and sees quality health care in promotion, preservation, and restoration. The interpretational or activity element is seen as meeting socially defined values and norms. Quality of care is thus seen as acceptable, pleasing and rewarding. Finally, the environmental element (an appropriately decorated room or a television) provides patient satisfaction and increases quality care through comfort, individuality, and security.

These basic elements offer a conceptual framework that helps define quality of care. However, we still need to define quality according to the situation in which we plan to assure its presence.

QUALITY ASSURANCE

The evolution of quality assurance has provided a multiplicity of definitions. However, within the long-term care facility, it is most commonly viewed as "a program designed to integrate existing mechanisms into a coordinated plan which assures high quality resident care. The quality of care is measured against standards set to achieve optimal results" (Greenblatt 1988).

With increased evidence that improved quality of care impacts the quality of life and maximizes the well-being of the health care recipient, quality assurance continues to flourish.

Although, ultimately, the impetus for quality assurance rests upon financial accountability, recreation professionals must also assume responsibility for the credibility and accountability of their programs. It therefore becomes the obligation (both morally and ethically) of the recreation professional to provide a service that influences the quality of life of the client. This service needs to be monitored through quality assurance, according to established standards.

Accountability to the administration and the board of directors of the long-term care facility is also necessary. This is accomplished, in part, by the ability to document positive changes in resident behavior or leisure lifestyle that are the result of the high level of activity programming.

Of equal importance, however, is accountability to clients themselves. Elderly residents of a nursing home are entitled to know what recreation services are available and how they might benefit from them.

However, the need to implement successful quality assurance programs, especially in recreation, are also due in part to factors beyond the control of the recreation or health care professional.

With the costs of long-term care reaching $76 billion by 1990 (Knight and Walker 1985) and with today's impending health care crises, emphasis on reimbursement rates has created an even greater reliance on regulatory agencies and their accreditation and survey processes. Today, in most instances, reimbursement rates are directly linked to the quality of services provided by the facility. Thus, now more than ever before, state health agencies have become the jury charged with evaluating the quality of care provided by long-term care facilities.

THE STATE SURVEY PROCESS: HISTORICAL PERSPECTIVES

In 1975, a resident of a Colorado nursing home sued the state for the lack of quality care she received. As a result, the state sued the federal government. With no system of survey in place and standards to be met, it was virtually impossible to determine what constituted quality of care. This case, Smith vs. Heckler, seemed to be the impetus for establishing criteria and standards that would be measured by the regulatory and accreditation agencies through their survey processes.

Through the second half of the 1970s, the survey process focused upon structural measures such as the presence of policies and procedures. This process was characterized by separate survey components (resident observation and PMR), which measured the facility's capabilities of providing care based on paper documentation. For recreation services, attendance statistics, progress reports, resident care plans and related documentation provided the proof of quality programming. The number of participants attending activities seemed to be more important than the appropriateness of the activities and the satisfaction of resident needs through available recreation programs.

In 1981, the implementation of the Sentinel Health Events (SHEs) provided the first outcome criteria that were utilized to identify and measure quality of care. The SHEs identified twelve areas of resident care that were intensely reviewed when their norms exceeded the predetermined threshholds (NYQAS Report #2). For recreation, residents were randomly selected for reviewing the presence of activities. This protocol established, for the first time, guidelines that determined whether appropriate recreation activities were planned and incorporated into the resident's daily program. Noninvolvement in activities presented a problem (i.e., SHE) if the resident's physical or mental health was at risk, if this was not a resident's choice, or if no evidence existed to support efforts by the activities staff to develop a plan of activities and encourage participation in the plan.

Since 1976, reimbursement rates for long-term care facilities have been linked in part to the New York State survey process. At that time, the federal government mandated that all states base their Medicaid reimbursement rates to facilities on the actual costs of running the facilities (PRI Reference Manual).

Increases were based upon the estimated inflation rate, with a ceiling set for cost containment. However, patient mix was not accounted for in reimbursement calculations, and all nursing homes received equal payment regardless of the level of care provided to their patients. As a result, many homes refused patients requiring heavier nursing care (Greenblatt 1988).

In 1983, the health care industry witnessed a revolutionary change. Resource Utilization Groups (RUGS), a new reimbursement rate system, were instituted in New York State. Initially, few probably realized the far-reaching effects RUGS would have on the survey process being implemented in New York State today.

Through the RUGS system, patients are classified into groups based upon similar clinical characteristics. The Patient Review Instrument (PRI) assesses patients according to categories, including behavioral problems, medical events, activities of daily living (eating, mobility, toileting and transfer), and specialized services such as occupational and physical therapy. The results of the PRI are reviewed periodically by nurse assessors to determine the level of care required by each patient. Thus, the case mix distribution of each facility now determines the reimbursement rate for that facility.

Through RUGS, documenting the kind of clinical care residents need becomes even more crucial for all disciplines, including recreation. For example, the resident who needs help with transferring in a wheel chair, assistance with eating, or help with toileting will presumably need this same assistance while at recreation programs (e.g., barbecues). Although in the past recreation therapists may have considered this a natural function of the job, RUGS now makes it necessary to document many of these events that indicate the type of care needed by the resident.

With the implementation of the SHEs and RUGS, yet another survey process was implemented in 1986. In place of the process that focused on structural measures such as the presence of policies and procedures, the long-term care survey focused on residents and the care they received (Balcerzak 1985). Thus, resident care became the significant issue, rather than paper work compliance with policies and procedures. Prior surveys found that paper work compliance did not necessarily equal quality care. In addition, certain facilities where structural requirements were not met seemed to provide quality care. Thus, the long-term care survey process known as the Patient Care and Service (PACS) process was instituted.

This survey, which became the foundation for NYQAS, consisted of four major activities: (1) in-depth, integrated, and resident-centered tour; (2) observation, interview, and resident review of in-depth sample of residents; (3) observation of drug pass; (4) observation of dining and eating (Balcerzak 1985).

The implications of PACS for recreation were significant and are still being felt. Residents are interviewed to determine if their recreation needs are met. In addition, activities are observed throughout the facility.

With the growing concern and increased significance of quality of care issues, the federal government mandated a quality assurance system in every long-term care facility. The New York State Quality Assurance System (NYQAS) was the result of the changing rationale in which past emphasis upon structural measures shifted to an even greater concern for quality care issues related to resident outcome.

In essence, NYQAS was made possible by a congruence of two events: "The development of the long-term care survey has created the structure for an outcome oriented approach, and the RUGS II data base has created a major outcome oriented data base" (NYQAS Report #2, p. 5).

Utilizing the RUGS II computerized case mix data base, NYQAS could target residents, which required reviews of specific clinical areas. Residents could therefore be reviewed for either improvements or deterioration in their functional abilities and limitations. In addition, NYQAS efficiently dealt with the negative incentives of RUGS. Any facility that allowed patients to deteriorate in hopes of receiving higher reimbursement rates was identified and cited by the NYQAS survey process.

With the advent of the Sentinel Health Events (SHEs) in 1981, twelve crucial outcome areas were reviewed to measure whether appropriate clinical care was available. In addition to these critical areas, residents were selected for interviews through the interview and record review system.

In NYQAS, CaRe groups replaced the twelve SHEs. Through the PRI data base, residents identified with potential problems in the

CaRe group areas were selected for in-depth interviews. Thus, the PRI is used to select residents based on the likelihood of a problem, and once the sample is selected, all residents in the sample receive an in-depth review. (NYQAS 1987). During the CaRe review, protocols developed for NYQAS that focus on quality of care were utilized. These specially designed protocols facilitate objective review of quality of care, which can be applied to long-term care facilities regardless of their location.

With the increased concern for quality of life issues and quality care, NYQAS built upon and enhanced the present long-term care survey, which affected the four major areas of the survey process.

Facility Tour. With the ability to focus upon potential problems identified by the PRI, the facility tour emphasizes areas not found on the PRI, including grooming, communication, and activities. With respect to these areas, problems related to quality of life are identified and reviewed in depth.

Drug Pass Observation. Distribution of medicine to residents continues to be observed. However, the PRI is able to target residents who may have problems with certain medications.

Observation, Interview, Record Review (OIRR). During the OIRR, observations were made throughout the facility and residents, families, and staff were interviewed. A review of areas such as activities, nutrition, rehabilitation, and activities of daily living helped determine whether resident needs were being met. Through the OIRR, NYQAS used CaRe groups to replace SHEs, in order to develop a broader base for review of quality of life issues.

Meal Observation. Finally, meal observation enabled NYQAS to determine if quality of life issues were being met in relation to nutritional needs, including parenteral or tube feeding.

The evolution of the state survey continues to unfold with yet another process, namely, the MDS (Minimum Data Set). This system represents, for the first time, a survey process based on standards set by the state and federal government.

The MDS, a client-centered approach, mandates a uniformed, consistent assessment of residents in every nursing home throughout the country. An integral piece of the MDS is the Comprehensive Care Plan written for the resident based on the information gathered by the professional in each discipline. Thus, the state survey process now focuses on the written care plan. Of equal importance is the need to implement each care plan, including evaluation and follow through.

IMPLICATIONS FOR THERAPEUTIC RECREATION

Providing quality therapeutic recreation services to the nursing home population can no longer rest upon certain "guidelines" whose principles are based on good intentions. A client-centered, systems approach must be provided upon which programs can be planned, implemented, and evaluated. Providing such an approach is essential for evaluating both the program and its effects upon client outcome.

Since NYQAS, quality of care issues continue to emerge as the focus in the provision of care. One of the most significant implications of NYQAS and the MDS lies in its recognition of the importance of the "social component" of care provided within the medical model still used by the long-term care facility. As Herb Shore (1986) notes:

> Much has been written about the medical model which generally implies the perception of the consumer of a human service as a 'sick patient,' who after 'diagnosis' is given 'treatment' for his or her 'disease,' by 'doctors' who carry primary administrative and human management responsibility and are assisted by a hierarchy of 'paramedical' personnel and 'therapists,' all this hopefully leading to a 'cure.' (p. 76)

As Shore agrees, medical care is important and has played a significant role in keeping the patient alive longer. However, as Shore suggested as far back as 1963,

> Long-term care facilities could establish their uniqueness and make a contribution to the field by focusing on the person (who might for a few hours be the patient) and on the fact that the social care philosophy permeated every fiber and sinew of long-term care programs and services, that social components

were a philosophical thrust, rather than being the assignment of a social worker or pastoral counselor. (p. 46)

With the heightened awareness that nursing homes are "homes" and the overemphasis of the medical model, the state and federal mandates have increasingly recognized the importance of recreation as a separate entity that impacts greatly upon the social care of the patient or resident. It therefore becomes the responsibility of the recreation professional to view the recent implementation of the MDS, not as another standard to be met, but rather, as the impetus to provide the highest level of quality programming possible.

Although the characteristics of the institutionalized aged have changed over recent years, the need to provide them with a meaningful program of recreation activities, regardless of their physical, psychological, or social limitations, remains the same. Thus, a crucial element in successful programming is our professional philosophy and our ability to maintain the "humanistic" value of the person we are serving. The medical and behavioral disorders, memory impairment, and social isolation often characteristic of the institutionalized elderly must not be a signal of automatic failure or inability to achieve some level of success in a recreation activity. Lack of opportunity for the institutionalized aged to satisfy their physical, cognitive, and affective needs through appropriate and meaningful recreation activities represents a basic disregard for the quality of care any human being is entitled to.

The health care professional can help add years to the life of the elderly. "Now we must work to ensure that quality is added to these years so that elders may not only live long but also well" (Shore 1986).

Through the provision of recreation as a human service element, we will hopefully achieve the highest level of quality care, which will ultimately help the elderly to "live well."

REFERENCES

Donabedian, A. 1978. "The Quality of Medical Care," *Science* 200 (May 26): 856-864.
Donabedian, A. 1968. "Promoting Quality Through Evaluating the Process of Patient Care," *Medical Care* 6.

Drude, K. and R. Nelson. 1982. "Quality Assurance: A Challenge for Community Health Centers." *Professional Psychology* 13(1): 85-90.

Balcerzak, S. 1985. "The Patent Care and Services (PACS) Survey, Update: The New Long-Term Care Survey Process," *The Journal of Long-Term Care Administration,* (Winter): 106-108.

Greenblatt, F. S. 1988. *Therapeutic Recreation for Long-Term Care Facilities.* New York: Human Sciences Press.

Havel, Z. 1981. "Quality of Care, Congruence, and Well-being Among Institutionalized Aged." *The Gerontologist* 14(1): 11-13.

Knight, B. and D. Walker. 1985. "Toward a Definition of Alternatives to Institutionalization for the Frail Elderly," *The Gerontologist* 15(4): 358-363.

Hammerman, J. 1974. "The Role of the Institution and the Concept of Parallel Services," *The Gerontologist* 14(1): 11-13.

New York Quality Assurance System. 1987. *Report 2. System Design: A Discussion of the NYQAS Survey Component.*

New York Office of Health System Management. *PRI Reference Manual: Long-Term Care Case Mix Reimbursement Project.*

Riley, B. 1987. "Conceptual Basis of Quality Assurance: Application to Therapeutic Recreation Service," *Evaluation of Therapeutic Recreation Through Quality Assurance.* State College, PA: Venture Publishing, pp. 7-21.

Shore, H. 1986. "Looking at Quality in Facility Living," *Provider* 4-8.

Wells, L. and C. Singer. 1988. "Quality of Life in Institutions for the Elderly: Maximizing Well Being," *The Gerontologist* 28(2): 266-269.

The Therapeutic Value of Art
for Persons
with Alzheimer's Disease
and Related Disorders

Jane E. Harlan

Six elderly persons are quietly working around a table. A woman is making a pastel drawing of the house and cherry tree she remembers from her childhood in Germany. A man paints a vase of daisies inspired by a still-life arrangement he is looking at, while another draws a portrait of the person sitting next to him. Some work with steady concentration; others forget to dip their brushes in the paint or can't remember what they were working on a moment before.

Scenes such as this have occurred every day as part of a model activity program established in New York City. Memory-impaired elders, who can be challenging to interest and sustain in active pursuits, became creatively engaged to an extent unexpected by the program staff. Group art therapy evolved into a unique and valued component of the program.

Art therapy is the use of painting, drawing, or sculpture by an individual to further his or her emotional and mental well-being. This takes place under the guidance of a professional trained in the use of art materials, in psychological functioning, and in therapeutic intervention. The American Art Therapy Association, founded in 1969, approves qualified training programs for art therapists, and establishes standards for the profession. Once most commonly found working in psychiatric units, art therapists now also provide

Jane E. Harlan is Research Associate, Indiana University, Institute for the Study of Developmental Disabilities, Bloomington, IN.

services in schools, senior centers, medical facilities, prisons, and many other settings.

The use of art as a treatment modality is based upon the healing qualities inherent in the art-making process. In using pencil, paint, or clay to make an image, we mobilize a complex combination of our emotional, intellectual, and manual faculties (Kramer, 1971). This process can facilitate the expression and integration of feelings and ideas to promote emotional growth, communication, and problem solving.

As in other creative arts modalities such as movement or music therapies, visual art expression offers an opportunity for nonverbal self-expression and the affirmation of the uniqueness of the individual through his or her creative endeavor. An environment is structured within which feelings, thoughts, and fantasies can be safely expressed. In music, movement, or art activities, there does not have to be a "right" or "wrong," and so there is less chance for experiencing failure.

The patient with Alzheimer's disease is faced with increasing confusion, declining self-esteem, and a fundamental loss of identity. For such individuals, the primary goals of art therapy treatment are: (1) to help preserve a sense of identity, (2) to facilitate the venting of emotions accompanying the disease process, so that remaining cognitive skills can be fully available, and (3) to counteract social isolation through sharing common concerns with peers. These goals are by necessity temporary due to the inevitable functional decline of persons with irreversible dementias.

Persons in the more advanced stages of dementia will probably be unable to use art materials (although they may frequently retain some capacity to be engaged by music). The basic skills required for painting are still accessible, however, to many of the mildly to moderately impaired. Because of the graphic qualities of the visual arts, art therapy is particularly suited for symbolic communication, and is especially rewarding in the tangible product that results.

Persons in the initial stages of dementia, who are aware of their losses but unable to function independently, are likely to resist participation in art groups if they perceive activities to be potentially infantilizing, unsuited to their experience, or revealing of embarrassing functional deficits. These fears can usually be alleviated by brief exposure to a well-designed program activity and the consistent presence of a reassuring staff member. Individual Alzheimer's patients and their families, too, appreciate the opportunity to be involved in pursuits that are age-appropriate and nondemeaning.

Art therapy can give the person with dementia an opportunity to express the overwhelming emotions that accompany devastating losses. It can provide a vehicle for reminiscence, reminding the individual of the higher functioning, accomplished person he or she once was. Continual decision making is required, engendering a sense of mastery. Structured creative activity that is challenging, but not threatening or overly-demanding, can help maintain some of the individual's sense of autonomy for a little longer. In addition, pride in the finished art work contributes to a sense of accomplishment and greater self-esteem.

Informal socialization inevitably unfolds during the working process, once the participants have achieved a feeling of secure belonging in the art group. Such spontaneous interaction is particularly important for persons with dementia, who face growing isolation as a result of diminished social competence, and stigmatization and fear on the part of friends, former co-workers and family. Group projects may also be devised that encourage greater interaction among the art therapy participants.

Wald (1986) has described the characteristics of art work by persons with dementia, emphasizing its simplicity, regression, disorganization, and confusion of perspective. Objects depicted may be fragmented, seen as parts rather than as a whole, or the images may lack boundaries separating one from another. Bizarre imagery such as fused animal and human figures may appear.

I discovered, however, that the art work of persons with Alzheimer's disease expresses the remaining strengths of the person creating it, in addition to the consequences of neurological deterioration. For example, one of my clients, a woman with Parkinson's disease, used pastels and paints to make works of great variety and intensity of color. Her art communicated the complex emotional vocabulary that could not be detected in her mask-like facial expression. A capacity for sensitivity was likewise apparent in the work of a man who was already quite impaired by Alzheimer's disease. His delicate lines and squiggles had a musical quality, simultaneously rhythmic and lyrical.

The art work of persons with dementia may also function for them as the positive attempt to cope with an environment which has become incomprehensible and frightening. Images associated with safety and enclosure, such as houses and containers, seemed frequently to be selected. One woman drew a house in a hurricane, saying, "It will survive; it's strong." Another clearly articulated her distress by creating a seascape in which drowning people cry out for help.

Art can be an important vehicle of communication for those who find verbal expression very stressful because of failing language capacities. The opportunity to say something without words, through line, form, and color, is often met with enthusiasm and relief. Persons experiencing immense losses are inevitably angry, despairing, or anxious. Their feelings may not be acceptable to family and other caregivers, or, indeed, to the client. A drawing, painting, or sculpture is a safe way to articulate and release these emotions (and may even be socially rewarded). Having such an outlet can make the individual's remaining cognitive resources more accessible so that he or she may function at the optimal level. For example, some relief from depression may cause a temporary recovery of some abilities that may have appeared to be permanently lost.

Clients welcome the opportunity to talk about their art work and their concerns. At our first meeting, a client told me through clenched teeth how angry she was, and that there was nothing she could do about it. I acknowledged her feelings. Later she seemed to take pleasure in using the art materials. She kissed my hand before leaving the room.

The inner experience of persons with Alzheimer's disease is difficult to gain access to because of the loss of language functions; art can provide a small window into this private world of suffering and bewilderment. The communicative function of art can assist those caring for the client to understand how he or she is perceiving and coping with the disease. What does the individual think is happening to him or her and why is it happening? For example, we might assume that the women who used the symbols of hurricanes and rough seas both felt ravaged by their losses, but that the one who said her house would survive the storm might be feeling less overwhelmed than the one who drew people drowning.

Clues to the meaning of the visual evidence (the art work) can be gained in observing and listening to the client while the art is being made, as well as in reviewing what is known about the person he or she used to be. An overlay of depression or psychosis may be discernible in the art of some persons with dementia (Wald 1989). Because the art therapist often works with a team of professionals, these observations can be shared and discussed with other staff to improve the quality of the care which is offered to the individual.

Memories may emerge graphically, when imagery is created, as well as through spontaneous verbal interchange within the art group. A process of life review through reminiscence has been recognized as an important feature of later life development for all persons (Butler 1963). Bringing past experience to awareness and transforming it into pictures and words can help temporarily to consolidate the sense of self that is being eroded by disease. It is particularly important for these individuals to be reminded of the higher levels of health and functioning they previously achieved. When one client was drawing hair, she began to talk about her former job as a beautician. A plain gray-painted background for a mural reminded another woman of "a fall evening, reading and eating a Mars bar."

Cherished independence is lost as self-care abilities decline. Supported creative art activities offer the opportunity for an increased sense of mastery. The art group participant gains a sense of control by manipulating the art materials as he or she wants and making decisions within a limited sphere. This may make adjustment to growing dependence in other areas more tolerable.

A man who had probably exercised a great deal of decision-making in his successful military career reacted to his growing losses with restlessness and frequent noncompliance with the routines of the day program. In the art room, he exhibited a contrasting engagement in his work and ability to concentrate for brief periods. In the context of art therapy, he was able to communicate the limits of the assistance he wished to accept from me. For example, when he finished one picture and was about to begin another, I suggested a new sheet of paper. He refused it and continued to draw on top of his first work. Respecting his wishes, I did not interfere. Eventually, too impaired to do art work, and incapable of participating in most program activities, he nevertheless was able to sit for relatively long periods looking at and talking about his portfolio of paintings and drawings.

Loss of autonomy is also frequently accompanied by lower self-esteem. Persons who were, until relatively recently, productive individuals, valued by co-workers, friends, or family, may feel worthless in the face of their illness. They may blame themselves for their inability to do what they used to do. Art work often seems to express feelings about the self, especially when human figures are depicted. One woman described her picture as "a little girl who was supposed to be a big girl." Another client labeled a male figure he had drawn as "a shrimp."

Clients frequently point out perceived shortcomings in their work, and may attempt to throw it away. A man who often referred to his picture as "a mish-mash" appeared to be expressing his feelings of frustration about his inability to think clearly as he once did. The art therapist's acceptance of critical comments such as these may help clients ventilate emotions relating to their losses. Clients may feel that their remaining capacities for judgment and discrimination are being recognized when their own negative appraisals of the art work are acknowledged. The client says, in effect, "I was once a person of greater accomplishments," and is not contradicted.

At the same time, with the support of the art therapist, the client learns to find unique aspects of the art work that can be valued, and by extension, comes to ascribe greater value to himself or herself. Self-critical remarks almost invariably decrease after a period of time within the group. Participants become less reluctant to sign their pictures, share them with others and display them on the wall. Positive comments about the efforts of others can be heard, frequently.

Because of the functional deficits of persons with Alzheimer's disease and related disorders, art activities must be designed carefully and extensive support by the art therapist may be required. Distractibility, restlessness, confusion, and vision difficulties necessitate a well-lit environment, free from glare and extraneous noises, which has been set aside exclusively for art therapy during the duration of the group. Art supplies must be simple to use and the table uncluttered. If white paper is used, it can be put on a working surface of color to minimize the difficulty of discriminating objects from their backgrounds.

Choices must be offered to counter passivity and make the activity meaningful for each person. The extent of the choice, however, will probably need to be limited to a greater or lesser degree (depending upon the needs of the individual) in order to prevent paralyzing anxiety or confusion. Breaking tasks down into component steps may make the difference between satisfaction and frustration. With these compensatory supports, participants in the art therapy group often show an appreciable improvement in concentration and length of attention span before further inevitable decline.

Creativity is enhanced when clients are able to work on individual pursuits that are suited to their interests, and to the level and type of functional abilities that remain. Groups of clients must be small. The frequent, active intervention of the art therapist will probably be necessary to get people started, particularly in the first weeks after they join the group. The ability to work independently grows as participants gain confidence in their work and realize that they don't need others' approval to initiate ideas. This independence is supported by the art therapist who provides stimulation (music, still-life objects to look at, touch, or smell, art reproductions), technical advice in how to use art materials, encouragement through observations of specific strengths noted in the work, and many other kinds of supportive interventions. This may include drawing examples of a few different ways to make trees, mixing a color the client describes, or putting a brush in the hand of someone who forgets to pick it up.

I have developed a series of "stimulus images" to help overcome the anxiety that may occur when confronting a blank, white, sheet of paper. The images, consisting of a few lines drawn by the art therapist, might suggest an idea for a design or specific image. They give the client who might otherwise be unable to work, a place to get started. The client may be offered a choice of several images which seem appropriate to his or her interests and artistic sensibility. Shapes of the stimulus images may be abstract or may suggest a person, house, vase, or other familiar figure. This kind of support allows clients to make a creative contribution when memory loss and fear of failure would otherwise inhibit such involvement. The results are quite varied, reflecting the unique qualities of the individual.

Group art projects are effective in enhancing motivation and confidence and overcoming isolation. In a cooperative endeavor, each person can make a special contribution while his or her shortcomings are minimized by the complementary abilities of others. A mural painting session can involve the highest functioning individuals in making people and similarly complex images, while others can be engaged in depicting sky, grass, snow, and backgrounds that demand less representational ability, yet require creativity in choice of color, brush strokes, and style.

Collaborative work on a life-size human figure drawing can strengthen a deteriorating sense of body image, explore sexual concerns, and provide a safe opportunity to create a picture of a person, a subject that many individuals with dementia are hesitant to tackle. A large abstract collage project of cut-out colored paper shapes removes the constricting perception that something has to "look like it's supposed to look." It also requires the group to make decisions together regarding the composition and placement of the shapes, working together toward a common goal.

Therapeutically supported creative art expression offers persons with dementia a challenging and stimulating experience, while not demanding more than that of which they are capable. These persons may possess, and perhaps share, a recovered memory, or a moment of beauty, humor, or insight. In this way, they gain an opportunity to hold on to part of themselves for a little while longer.

REFERENCES

Butler, R. 1963. "The Life Review: An Interpretation of Reminiscence in the Aged." *Psychiatry, Journal for the Study of Interpersonal Processes,* 26.

Kramer, E. 1971. *Art As Therapy with Children.* New York: Schocken Books.

Wald, J. 1989. "Art Therapy for Patients with Alzheimer's Disease and Related Disorders." In H. Wadeson, J. Durkin, and D. Perach (eds), *Advances in Art Therapy,* New York: John Wiley & Sons.

Wald, J. 1986. "Fusion of Symbols, Confusion of Boundaries: Percept Contamination in the Art Work of Alzheimer's Disease Patients." *Art Therapy* 3 (2), pp. 74-80.

The Effectiveness of Cueing
on Anagram Solving by Cognitively
Impaired Nursing Home Elderly

Kestal T. Phillips

Mental status tests used to assess cognitive impairment in the elderly may give too narrow a representation of their cognitive abilities. Consequently, recreational programming for the demented elderly could be negatively influenced by such test results. A bias exists against programming challenging intellectual activities. Poor performance on a mental status test may not reliably predict a patient's capacity to participate successfully in recreational activities, such as word games, that primarily involve decision-making and problem-solving skills. Recreation therapists need to research specific strategies that enable patients' cognitive functioning and recreational participation. Toward that end, the present study investigated the relationship between cueing with taxonomic category labels and the anagram-solving performance of elderly individuals impaired with irreversible dementia.

HYPOTHESES

Anagrams of taxonomic category instances were presented to cognitively impaired elderly in noncued and cued game formats. It was hypothesized that cueing with taxonomic category labels would increase subjects' total number of correct answers to one-word,

Kestal T. Phillips, MS, is Supervisor, Crises Intervention Hotline, Chapel Hill, NC.

one-solution anagrams compared to a noncued condition. Individual and group performance levels were expected to improve under cued conditions. A second hypothesis predicted that cueing with taxonomic category labels would reduce individual and group anagram solution times compared to a noncued condition.

DEFINITION OF TERMS

Anagram: a word puzzle consisting of scrambled letters which, when correctly rearranged, spell a single word.

Taxonomy: the systematic classification of items with regard to their natural relationships.

Cue: the name of the taxonomic category from which an anagram's solution word was selected, verbally communicated to subjects by the researcher.

Cognitively impaired elderly: nursing home residents diagnosed with a dementia of the Alzheimer's type, organic brain syndrome, or organic mental syndrome whose score on a selected mental status test indicated the presence of cognitive deficits.

REVIEW OF THE LITERATURE

No anagram studies with dementia patients as subjects were encountered in the literature. Studies involving nondemented subjects (Schuberth, Spoehr and Haertel 1979; Richardson and Johnson 1980; Seidenstadt 1982) have demonstrated that anagram solving is facilitated by the presentation of category-label cues. Dominowski and Ekstrand (1967) found that direct and associative priming increased the availability of possible solution words to subjects, which facilitated decreased anagram solution times.

Investigators have examined the impact of cueing on the cognitive functioning of aged dementia patients. Miller (1975), and Morris, Wheatley, and Britton (1983) found that the presentation of letter cues resulted in no significant difference between the cued recall performance of dementia patients and nondemented controls.

Evidence obtained by Diesfeldt (1985) supported his hypothesis that senile dementia does not so much impair category knowledge as category retrieval. He suggested that the impoverished speech in dementia may be explained as diminished access to certain words rather then as the permanent loss of words and their meanings from the patient's vocabulary. Diesfeldt's dementia subjects were better able to correctly recognize exemplars of different categories than to generate examples from memory. They possessed enough knowledge of the generalized attributes of an item to recognize it as belonging to a specified category.

Some researchers have argued that cues alone cannot enhance the memory functioning of dementia patients. Davis and Mumford (1984) compared memory performance for word lists between persons with an Alzheimer's-type dementia and unimpaired controls. Letter cueing facilitated the performance of dementia subjects, but the increase in recall did not exceed that of the controls. Category cueing did not produce significantly better performance than non-cued recall for the dementia patients. Hanley (cited in Davis and Mumford) studied aspects of reality orientation therapy with hospitalized dementia patients. Retrieval prompts (signs and signposts) alone did not improve the word orientation of the patients, but such aids combined with an active word orientation training program did. Diesfeldt (1984) asked institutionalized persons with Alzheimer's-type dementia to learn a categorized word list under different encoding and retrieval conditions. Recall was best when an explanation of the category structure accompanied cueing with category names at recall. Information about the category structure did not by itself increase recall, nor did only the presentation of category-name cues at the time of recall.

An explanation for memory dysfunction in dementia is controversial. Conclusions drawn by some investigators have supported the retrieval-deficit hypothesis, while others have argued that dementia impairs the ability to process, code, and store information in memory, as well as retrieval mechanisms. Cues have assisted the demented elderly with memory tasks. Some researchers have suggested that the effectiveness of cueing on memory dysfunction in the elderly may depend on the amount and kind of information to be remembered, types of cues and presentation conditions, and the presence or absence of reinforcement techniques such as behavioral training.

METHODS

Subjects

Thirteen residents (mean age 85.6 years) from three nursing homes in the New York City area participated in the study. Diagnostic information was obtained from each subject's medical chart. Seven persons were free of cardiovascular disease, and the dementia diagnoses for the group were as follows: five SDAT (senile dementia of the Alzheimer's type), one OBS (organic brain syndrome) and one OMS (organic mental syndrome). Six others had cardiovascular disease with the following dementia diagnoses: two AD (Alzheimer's disease), one SDAT, one OBS, one OBS with myocardial infarction and cerebrovascular insufficiency, and one OMS. Persons with a history of substance abuse or seizures were excluded. Medications were not controlled. The six-item Orientation-Memory-Concentration Test (Katzman, Brown, Fuld, Peck, Schechter, and Schimmel 1983) was administered to potential subjects to help differentiate among mild, moderate, and severe cognitive deficits. Persons scoring from 10 to a maximum of 28 points were eligible, provided they demonstrated comprehension of the concept of anagram solving and an ability to follow verbal instructions. The Katzman scores of the 13 subject ranged from 10 to 28. These scores indicated that one subject was minimally impaired, nine moderately so, and three had severe cognitive impairment.

Anagram Materials and Apparatus

Each anagram was a word puzzle consisting of five scrambled letters which, when correctly rearranged, spelled a single, five-letter, English word. A different anagram letter order was randomly assigned to each of the eight solution words. The letter orders were among those suggested by Dominowski (1966). An anagram required either one, two, or three letter moves for solution. No anagram letter order began with the initial letter of the solution word.

The solution words were exemplars selected from eight semantically unrelated categories in the Battig and Montague (1969) norms. These solution words were matched against a list of single-solution, five-letter words compiled by Olson and Schwartz (1967). The cue for each anagram was the name of the taxonomic category from which its solution word was drawn. Instance dominance refers to how frequently a particular response is given as an exemplar of a category. Solution words with a medium instance-dominance rank (Schuberth et al. 1979) were used; that is, each solution word ranked between 7 and 19 in its respective category in the Battig and Montague norms. Words that were not the most common associates of their respective categories were selected to decrease the probability that correct answers were simply random guesswork by subjects.

Each anagram was stencilled in uppercase, block letters 10mm high on a separate sheet of white bristol board (28 × 36mm). Letters were written in black felt pen. Each anagram card was placed on a desktop bookstand for viewing by the subjects. A stopwatch was used to measure solution times. Responses and times were recorded on individual data sheets.

Design and Procedure

No models of anagram solution with dementia patients as subjects were found in the literature. The experiment was a one-group, pretest-posttest design, and was modeled after anagram studies conducted by Schuberth et al. (1979) and Richardson and Johnson (1980). Thirteen subjects were tested individually. They were asked to solve the same set of eight anagrams with and without category-label cues. A period of seven to ten days separated the two presentation conditions. The sequence of the noncued and cued conditions was counterbalanced across subjects. Anagrams were presented one at a time. Subjects were told that each anagram had but one solution, which was a word in the English language. A correct response was exact pronunciation of the solution word. Maximum allowable solution time was 100 seconds. Instructions and cues were repeated at 30-second intervals. Solutions were given verbally. No writing materials were used by subjects. Solution times to the nearest one-tenth of a second were measured by stopwatch and recorded. Upon solution or expiration of the time limit, the next anagram was presented after a pause of 15 seconds. In the noncued game, subjects only recalled verbal instructions to rearrange the letters on each card to make one English word. In the cued game, the verbal instructions were accompanied by a category-label cue for each anagram.

RESULTS AND INTERPRETATION OF FINDINGS

The 13 subjects' scores on a mental status test (Katzman et al. 1983) suggested that 12 of them had either moderate or severe cognitive impairment, yet each subject solved at least one noncued anagram, and seven individuals solved four or more of eight noncued anagrams. Table 1 indicates that a high Katzman score (20 or above), indicating severe impairment, did not necessarily predict a poor performance, nor did the lowest Katzman score of 10 correlate with an exceptionally good performance. Eight subjects were diagnosed with an Alzheimer's-type dementia. Five of them solved four or more noncued anagrams despite Katzman scores above 20. This is a surprising finding, given the impoverished vocabulary and word-finding difficulties commonly reported in persons with an Alzheimer's-type dementia (Appell, Kertesz, and Fisman 1982). The fact that several subjects succeeded in solving anagrams without cues challenges the typically low expectations that caregivers exhibit about the decision-making and problem-solving capabilities of elderly dementia patients.

With cueing, every subject equalled or improved his or her noncued solution score. Eleven individuals solved one to five more anagrams when cued with taxonomic category labels. As a group, subjects solved an additional 29 items when cued, which resulted in a group improvement rate of 58%.

As seen in Table 2, the cued group solution score was superior to the noncued group solution score for each of the eight anagrams. The group improvement factor ranged from one to seven anagrams additionally solved under cued conditions. The hypothesis that cueing with taxonomic category labels would increase subjects' total number of correct answers to one-word, one-solution anagrams

TABLE 1
INDIVIDUAL KATZMAN SCORE AND COMPARISON OF
INDIVIDUAL NONCUED AND CUED SOLUTION SCORES

Subject ID#	Katzman Score	Noncued Score	Cued Score	Improvement Factor
01	28	5	5	0
02	21	4	7	3
03	17	4	6	2
04	24	1	3	2
05	24	6	7	1
06	22	2	4	2
07	10	3	7	4
08	21	2	7	5
09	22	2	6	4
10	22	7	7	0
11	21	2	5	3
12	14	7	8	1
13	17	5	7	2
Total:		50	79	29

Note: Numerals in the noncued and cued solution score columns indicate the total number of anagrams solved out of 8. Improvement factor is the additional number of anagrams solved by each subject in the cued game. Zero (0) in that column means cued/noncued scores were identical.

compared to a noncued condition was supported for 11 of 13 individuals and for the group as a whole.

It was hypothesized that cueing with taxonomic category labels would reduce individual and group anagram-solution times compared to a noncued condition. Group mean times were reduced for five of the eight anagrams under cued conditions. Five of 13 individuals had shorter cued than noncued mean times. However, the eight subjects whose cued mean times were longer than their noncued mean times solved more anagrams when cued. The fact that cueing with taxonomic category labels did not reduce individual solution times for the majority of subjects is not necessarily a negative finding. Cues may have triggered an intensified search and retrieval process. Subjects might have utilized the cues to conduct a more deliberate and specific cognitive search than was possible under noncued conditions when responses may have been more intuitive. A striking contrast between the noncued and cued ana-

TABLE 2
COMPARISONS OF NONCUED AND CUED
GROUP SOLUTION SCORES BY ANAGRAM

Anagram	Solution	Noncued Group Score	Cued Group Score	Group Improvement
REDSS	DRESS	8	12	4
TMUHO	MOUTH	4	6	2
PNAAJ	JAPAN	8	10	2
IENCE	NIECE	6	11	5
OESUM	MOUSE	0	5	5
IONNO	ONION	5	12	7
OBNAJ	BANJO	9	10	1
HCOUC	COUCH	10	13	3

Note: Group solution scores refer to how many of 13 subjects solved a specific anagram under noncued and cued conditions. Group improvement indicates the additional number of subjects who solved a specific anagram in the cued game compared to the noncued game.

gram-solving performances was the number of different incorrect answers the subjects proposed. A total of 105 different incorrect answers were proposed in the noncued game, compared to only 35 in the cued game. Perhaps subjects' thinking was more specifically directed by cues, and evaluation of an answer in relation to a cue before articulating it might have occurred.

The anagram-solving performance of all subjects improved with the presentation of taxonomic category-label cues. Individuals either solved more anagrams, reduced their solution times, or both, when cued. The results suggest that in elderly persons impaired with irreversible dementia, cueing was an enabling strategy that helped direct and enhance cognitive functions required to solve anagrams. All subjects said they believed the cues were helpful, and some articulated more specifically that cueing either directed or quickened their thinking. Clients' belief that cueing is enabling has important clinical implications. If they associate cues with increased effectiveness of personal responses, their interest, involvement, and success in recreational activities that employ cueing strategies may increase, and self-esteem may be enhanced. Subjects expressed surprise at their ability to solve anagrams and were pleased with their success.

In this study, elderly nursing home residents impaired with irreversible dementia demonstrated the ability to solve noncued and cued anagrams. This suggests that elderly dementia patients are capable of more effortful, sophisticated cognitive processing involving semantic information than is generally believed. Subjects had no previous experience solving anagrams but retained the game concept well and succeeded, which implies an ability to learn and participate in recreational activities that are new, verbal, and intellectually challenging. It is hoped that the information and conclusions summarized in this chapter will prompt recreation therapists to question any negative biases that may unnecessarily restrict their programming options for elderly dementia patients. Cueing appears to be a viable intervention that can enhance these patients' cognitive functioning and recreational participation.

LIMITATIONS

There was a heterogeneity of dementia diagnoses among the small sample of subjects. While this fact cautions against generalization of the findings, the researcher believes the evidence indicates that anagram programming is a therapeutic activity for elderly persons with dementia. The application of cueing techniques in word game programming and other recreational activities for the demented elderly deserves further study. Future anagram research should involve larger and homogeneous sample groups, stricter diagnostic criteria, randomization in sampling, and uniform testing conditions.

REFERENCES

Appell, J., A. Kertesz, and M. Fisman. 1982 "A Study of Language Functioning in Alzheimer Patients." *Brain and Language* 17:73-91.

Battig, W., and W. Montague. 1969. "Category Norms for Verbal Items in 56 Categories: A Replication and Extension of the Connecticut Category Norms." *Journal of Experimental Psychology Monographs* 80(3) Pt. 2.

Davis, P., and S. Mumford. 1984. "Cued Recall and the Nature of the Memory Disorder in Dementia." *British Journal of Psychiatry* 144:383-386.

Diesfeldt, H. 1984. "The Importance of Encoding Instructions and Retrieval Cues in the Assessment of Memory in Senile Dementia." *Archives of Gerontology and Geriatrics* 4:231-239.

Dominowski, R., and B. Ekstrand. 1967. "Direct and Associative Priming in Anagram Solving." *Journal of Experimental Psychology* 74:84-87.

Katzman, R., T. Brown, P. Fuld, A. Peck, R. Schecter, and H. Schimmel. 1983. "Validation of a Short Orientation-Memory-Concentration Test of Cognitive Impairment." *American Journal of Psychiatry* 140:734-739.

Miller, E. 1975. "Impaired Recall and Memory Disturbances in Presenile Dementia." *British Journal of Social and Clinical Psychology* 14:73-79.

Morris, R., J. Wheatley, and P. Britton. 1983. "Retrieval from Long-term Memory in Senile Dementia: Cued Recall Revisited." *British Journal of Clinical Psychology* 22:141-142.

Olson, R., and R. Schwartz. 1967. "Single and Multiple Solution Five-letter Words." *Psychonomic Monograph Supplements* 2(8):105-151.

Richardson, J., and P. Johnson. 1980. "Models of Anagram Solution." *Bulletin of the Psychonomic Society* 16(4):247-250.

Schuberth, R., K. Spoehr, and R. J. Haertel. 1979. "Solving Anagrams: Category Priming and the Differential Availability of Category Solutions." *Quarterly Journal of Experimental Psychology* 31:599-607.

Seidenstadt, R. 1982. "Category Label and List-item Priming in Anagram Solving." *Psychological Reports* 51:207-211.

Recreation in the Nursing Home

Elaine Streitfeld

For 18 years, I was supervisor of arts and crafts at the Hebrew Home for the Aged in Riverdale, New York. Here, with seven staff members, I taught various crafts to the 70 residents who came daily to the Arts and Crafts room.

We worked with a wide range of residents, some needing minimal assistance, others who were very ill, some with Alzheimer's disease or related disorders. Each resident had a choice of painting, sculpture, ceramics, knitting, crocheting, sewing, rug-weaving, mosaics, or making enamelled jewelry. Our goals were to design and create programs to fit the special needs of our clients–to help them transcend the often painful and negative aspects of aging and institutional living.

I learned how important autonomy was and offered the residents activities that enabled them to make their own decisions. I wanted them to enjoy the time they spent doing work that was not just busy work, but that provided them with satisfying and gratifying experiences. To have them feel comfortable and secure in my presence was my desire. I also wanted to encourage interaction and provide stimuli for socialization, in an atmosphere where their efforts were respected and appreciated.

In teaching art, the essence is the commitment and courage of each individual to say something in a way that only he or she can. For this, it is important to impart the feeling of serenity that some of them had lost in coming into the institution.

Since living in a special setting for the elderly is serious business, as is the aging process, I learned that fun and frequent celebrations

Elaine Streitfeld is Supervisor of Arts and Crafts, Hebrew Home and Hospital for the Aged, Bronx, NY.

were quite valuable. Twice a year, during the spring and winter, we had parties in the arts and crafts program. A resident committee decided on a delicious menu that differed from their regular fare. Our staff took great pains to decorate the room in a festive manner. Over a hundred residents attended, folk singers entertained, and certificates of appreciation were given to participants in the program.

To make the parties more festive, we chose special themes. These included a grape festival, a Japanese garden, and an African festival where we honored staff members who came dressed in their native African costumes. We also had frequent parties to celebrate all happy events with staff and residents sharing joy together.

One of the most difficult problems we faced was the negative feelings and depression of residents. Sometimes it felt as if we were pushing a heavy stone uphill. Admission trauma was frequent with our clients, and the sense of self-esteem was low. We learned to persist when faced with refusal to participate, realizing that fear of failure was an important part of negative response.

One of our clients, Dr. S., was a tall, aristocratic, elegant man who had a profound hearing loss, which isolated him from his peers. He was an intellectual who quoted Socrates and Shakespeare from memory. Anxious to involve him in painting, I asked him if he had ever done any art work. He replied, "Yes, but I was dissatisfied with the poor results." I sensed he was interested, but unsure. Handing him canvas, brushes, and helping him get started by squeezing out all the wonderful, seductive colors, I said with a welcoming smile, making eye contact, "Sit down here and just enjoy mixing some colors" (a non-threatening directive).

Dr. S. became addicted to painting. He came every day and with serious intent completed one fine canvas after another. He even had three one-man shows! In a few years he had developed a style of his own, and won prizes for his beautiful landscapes. He began to communicate a sense of pride and a belief in his artistic ability. His paintings became his connection to people and his hearing loss no longer isolated him as it had. He once told me, "I dream painting. I wish I had become an artist instead of a doctor."

His paintings often indicated how he felt. His first one was of a tiny tree bent over in a winter forest. It stood alone and sad, just as he felt when he first entered the home. Later, with his confidence returning because of the approval he was getting, he painted another tree in a winter forest, but this one seemed strong. It was standing upright with its branches outstretched and reaching. He had found his raison d'être and now felt comfortable enough to reach out to those around him.

Shortly afterward, he suffered a stroke. When I visited him, he told me, "I don't know if I'll be able to paint again." I encouraged him by saying, "You'll never know unless you try." To our mutual amazement, he was able to paint by supporting his weak brush hand with his strong left hand. He painted his stroke as a falling tree in that same winter forest which symbolized his old age. Later, he painted a self-portrait–a strong old gnarled tree with many dead branches, but there were also branches with brightly colored autumn leaves on them. He said of this painting, "This tree is old and dying, but, look, there is still life in it." Dr. S. taught me how important self-expression is, and how healing it can be.

Many of the residents at the home feel abandoned by their children who do not visit them as often as they would like. Others have difficulty socializing because they are often depressed. To give them a haven to share their feelings and experiences, I formed the "Tea and Conversation Group."

This group consisted of approximately 20 people meeting weekly to say what was on their minds and discuss topics they felt were pertinent to their lives. Topics included sex, death, politics, self-comfort, their children, and self-assertiveness. We had three sessions on this last topic with an expert from the Riverdale Mental Health Clinic. Often the residents would speak on subjects on which they had expertise.

One fascinating session included discussion of how they felt about being old. The descriptions used were: peaceful, tolerant, understanding, accepting, submitting, wise, regretful, boring, loving, fearful, angry, sick, successful, grateful, and appreciated. One woman said, "I'm lucky to have reached this stage and seen a complete cycle." Another said, "I learned to accept and cope." Others found that they were at peace, and happy they did not have the burdensome responsibilities of earlier years.

In a home for the aged, the subjects of sex and death are taboo.

These were brought up by the group and discussed, much to the relief of some of the residents. An unusual feeling of trust was established so that one of the group was able to confide that she had attempted suicide prior to her admission to the home. My role in the group was facilitator, trying to encourage the shy, introverted people in the group to express their opinions. Often, members of the group became rude and intolerant when unpopular viewpoints were expressed. I reminded them that everyone's view was important. The Tea and Conversation group still meets. It seems to fill the need in residents' lives of ventilating their anxieties and fears. It also serves as a place where one can laugh and cry.

For many years the one-person art exhibits were very popular. In an institutional setting where one eats and celebrates one's birthday in groups, I felt that the individual residents should be singled out for recognition for their creative efforts.

Once a month, flyers announcing a one-person exhibit were sent to staff, residents, and relatives. The honored individual's work was hung with care. Refreshments were served, speeches were made by both staff and residents praising the work. What they had made with their hands and mind was important and beautiful, and we told them so.

One woman who had done very exciting paintings walked to the place of honor in a chiffon dress and had a proud smile on her face. She told me later, that day was almost as important to her as her wedding day.

Art films were shown as part of our program. The one-person exhibit was an ego-building experience which reinforced feelings of self-worth. Each person cherished the feeling of being singled out and appreciated. For each artist, it was a day to be remembered and for their children it was a special gift to see their parents in a new light–vital, creative, and alive.

Creativity is the ability to see things in a new way; to recognize what is significant; to relate meaningful observations, and to pull them together into some new whole. I had the privilege of knowing a person with just such gifts at the home. Elsie had never painted before she came into the home, but learned fast and found much joy in it.

She had written, "Since I've started painting, a new and beautiful world has opened before my eyes. I can thrill to the melodious song of birds, and find beauty in their multi-colored plumage. Every blade of grass has meaning to me. Pebbles and rocks enthrall me. The constantly changing color of the sky, the changing forms of the clouds, and the interesting shapes of the trees are so wondrous to behold."

Meditation was introduced to the residents when the home started a wellness program and asked me to form and lead a group. I had been meditating for five years, and was happy to share what I had learned. Thirty people came to the initial session. To set the proper spiritual atmosphere, I covered the table with an ancient Japanese obi, a vase containing a rose, some seagull feathers, pebbles from a beach, and lighted candles. I had no idea how the residents would respond, and was amazed at how receptive they were to this new experience.

I dimmed the lights, and began the session by asking them to smell the rose, touch the feathers and pebbles to give them a connection to nature. The stressful conditions of their lives made them focus on their illnesses and losses. To help them learn to relax and to let go of destructive thoughts, I took them on a "guided fantasy." Later I asked them to go to their own special place where they felt safe and comfortable. They each had wonderful experiences that seemed to promote peace, calm, and healing. I took notes on some of the comments residents made concerning the benefits they experienced through the meditation.

L. said, "The rock was warm on my back. It felt so nice and comfortable that I dropped into a void. Tears came to my eyes. I didn't want to move." M. said, "I had a pain in my shoulder, and when I meditated, it sent a healing rainbow there. The area became warm, and the pain disappeared." H. said, "It was like a dream. I was floating our of my body." N. commented, "I felt empty. I emptied myself and I became hollow."

I had honestly expected much more resistance. Many of them had never heard of meditation, and came to the group simply because they trusted me. I presented it as a tool they could use in their lives to alleviate stress, help them heal themselves, and give them serenity. This was indeed a tall order, but their comments were positive, and their continued attendance twice a week attested to the benefits they derived.

I also used meditation with the high-functioning Alzheimer's patients. In the guided fantasy, I took them on a calm lake in a boat. I told them the sun shone overhead and a soft breeze caressed their faces. I stressed the safety of the boat. Some of the patients kept their eyes closed. Others fell asleep. I always told the people who fell asleep they were *really* relaxing to spare them embarrassment. With the Alzheimer's patients, the boat ride always brought back memories and stories of the boat trips they had enjoyed in their early years.

To attract new residents to the arts and crafts program, we arranged "happenings." A guest portrait artist came to paint portraits of the residents in watercolor. Slides of trips to China and India were shown as well as colorful folk art collected on these trips. We also gave workshops to introduce new crafts. These were experimental, and included such topics as working with clay, how to make greeting cards, how to batik cloth and make scarves, and how to paint T-shirts. Attendance was often high at the happenings, and new skills were learned.

When S. completed her colorful wall hanging of Noah's Ark, she decided to give it to the Ittleson School, a nearby residence for emotionally disturbed children. That was the beginning of many intergenerational programs I was to lead. Later, the Bronx Council on the Arts gave us funds to continue this very worthwhile exchange between young and old. Many murals were created by the group. One was given to St. Joseph's Hospital and placed in their emergency room; another was given to a child abuse center, and a third was given to the Richmond Center, a home for profoundly handicapped children.

All the sites were chosen by the residents and the children. The institutions showed their appreciation by inviting the children and residents to ceremonies dedicating the murals. While members of the press took photos, a good time was had by all. This gave both groups a sense of great accomplishment and joy. For the elderly, it was a connection with the outside world.

Relationships were formed and creative juices flowed, as did the love and friendships. One of the residents observed, "Mothers today do not have the time and energy to give to their children, since they work all day." They felt they were fulfilling an important need, as indeed they were. For the children, a great many stereotypical images of the elderly were dispelled, and feelings of genuine warmth and trust emerged.

One exciting collaboration was on the Peace Project. It had begun out of a discussion about peace. The two groups wanted to know what they could do to promote peace. Somebody suggested writing letters to President Reagan, Premier Gorbachev, and the U.N. So, letters were written to these world leaders, asking for peaceful solutions to international problems. They were assembled in the form of a peace scroll and decorated with paintings and collages. Rep. Ted Weiss accepted the responsibility of taking the scroll to Washington to give to the President, who sent a reply. There was a moving ceremony at the U.N. where the peace bell was rung and where the scroll still hangs.

Each experience I led was rewarding, but the one which combined 11-year-olds and Alzheimer's patients was the most challenging. The children had been briefed in simple terms about the nature of the disease and some possible problems they might encounter. We had to deal with the fears of children upon seeing adults in confused and often helpless states. We told them that some of the patients would be unable to speak.

I asked them how they would communicate with the Alzheimer's patients. One child said, "I can smile at them." Another responded with, "I could touch them in a gentle way." These were, of course, excellent approaches and in practice elicited positive responses from the patients. At the end of the program, I asked the children what they thought of their experience. They were able to speak of their anxieties and fears in dealing with confused and nonverbal patients. Most of them felt good about being in a position of giving to adults. As one child put it, "Grown-ups usually do things for us. It felt good giving to them for a change."

As the program progressed, the residents began to complain that the intergenerational meetings interfered with their work in arts and crafts. When the children came, they had to stop what they were doing. While I could certainly understand why they wanted to finish what they were doing, I also had seen the expressions of joy on their faces when the children entered the room.

I asked them if teenagers might be more stimulating to work

with, and some residents agreed to work with gifted teenagers from DeWitt Clinton High School. A musical fashion show was chosen for this project, and I worked closely with those who wrote the narration and designed the costumes. When the script was completed, they designed imaginative costumes and proudly performed together.

While working with Alzheimer's patients, I did background on the disease and its treatment. I was surprised to discover in the literature little reference to activities that might be appropriate for my clients. I realized that the patients with whom I worked had distinct needs different from those of the well aged. Aware of their limitations, I tried a number of new approaches in designing programs for them. Usually we gathered in a circle. Some were only moderately impaired, while others were more regressed. Although the latter group did not seem to respond, they enjoyed being part of the group.

Moving to music gave them a great deal of enjoyment. As a variation on this activity, I constructed a maypole with brightly colored ribbons attached to it. The ends of the ribbons were held by the residents (especially meaningful for wheelchair residents, as it made them connected to the group). Using lively music, I showed them how to wave, wriggle, and ripple the colored bands to keep in time with the music.

When I realized how much the patients needed and desired affection, I designed the "hugging doll." It is about four feet tall, large and soft. Once the doll was stitched up, I had the patients participate in deciding about the features. Should they be smiling or sad? What color should the hair be? More decisions were required to determine the sex of the doll, the kind of clothing. The finished doll was passed around for everyone to hug. J. put it on his knee and gave it a ride; S. cradled it in her arms and sang it a lullaby. They gave the doll a name, and the patient who had chosen a lucky number got to keep it. I made new dolls until all the patients had their own.

Puppets are also lots of fun, and a way to relate to the patients. Often, patients who would not respond to me, reacted to the puppet. Since families are important, I made a family of them for their dramatic play. There was a mother with wrinkles, dressed attractively, with pearls. I'd ask them, "Why does mother have wrinkles?

What sort of work does she do?" The father had a tweed suit, red tie, and a moustache; the little girl had red pigtails and a smile, and her brother had tears falling on his cheeks. When I asked them to explain the tears, they would say, "Nobody comes to visit him," or "the food is bad." They also requested a grandmother and grandfather puppet, as well as a baby and a family dog. We had wonderful moments creating scenes for the family. Sometimes it was a picnic, wedding, family fight, or a honeymoon. They took part by choosing a character they wished to represent, and often replayed stories from their own past lives.

Experience taught me that I could be more effective becoming part of the group. They would then imitate my behavior, and paint, dance, act, or talk of their own feelings. I was the leader as well as one of the group.

The rhythmic quality of poetry and its similarity to music produces a response in those who have sensory deficits. The cadence of poetry proved to be soothing and comforting, while the words stimulated discussion and peer interaction.

I set a large pad on an easel and put out watercolors. I would then recite Haiku poetry. I used Haiku because it presented simple images with which they would have no difficulty relating. For example:

> Butterfly floats through air
> Cloudy autumn sky.

Or,

> Seagulls flying
> Over ruined sand castles
> Carried by the wind.

The patients were then asked what they would like me to paint—What color should it be? Where was it to be placed? At times, they took brush in hand and painted the wind or the seagull.

The goals I had with the Alzheimer's patients were to provide them with opportunities to be successful, to let them experience quality time together, as well as to focus on their prevailing strengths. It is important to realize that, despite their many cognitive losses, there are great affective resources within these patients. I have found that recreation can make these resources available to them. Through the creative arts, social celebrations, discussions, and meditation, people are freed, in a way, from their limitations, and enabled to experience a richer life. There is a quality of transcendence in leisure that permits us to go beyond ourselves. This is what I learned from my work with the elderly.

Playing for Keeps

Michael Spiegel

My world is a very private world, usually reserved for just my patients and myself, but, for today, I am going to invite you into my world, the world of a therapeutic recreation professional on an acute psychiatric ward, where life and death literally hang in the balance, and where, as therapeutic recreation practitioners, we are, indeed, playing for keeps.

In 1977 I met a patient named L. She was very, very nervous, agitated, and actively suicidal. Only 18 years of age, her mother and father had both died shortly before her admission to the hospital. She clearly did not want to live, and her agitation caused her to stutter uncontrollably. She would walk around trying to remove an imaginary knife which she believed to be stuck in her neck. With great difficulty I persuaded her to come to my music therapy group. In this group, I play the guitar and patients participate as they are able to–watching, listening, tapping, clapping, playing an instrument, singing. For the first two or three days that she attended, L. only sat and stared. By week's end, I noticed her feet tapping lightly to the beat of "He's got the whole world in his hands." During the second week she started clapping. Then, in the middle of the third week, she was reading from a song book, which she asked to borrow before the group got started. After four weeks, L. stood up in the group, walked over to me, took the song book out of my hands, gently, but with authority, and said "Mike, that's not how it goes. Here, let me show you."

Shortly after that, L. and I started an international folk dance class for all other patients to learn Mexican, Greek, Russian, Ser-

Michael Spiegel, MS, is Director of Activity Therapy, Lincoln Hospital Mental Health Center, Bronx, NY.

127

bian, Israeli, and American folk dances. Later, more and more patients became involved, but L. was always the leader, with me, instructing the other patients and directing the group.

In 1980, L. called me from Brooklyn. I hadn't seen or heard from her since her discharge. She informed me that she was completing her degree in therapeutic recreation. She asked my help in her preparation for taking the state exam in therapeutic recreation, which she passed, and then later, when preparing for job interviews. She was successful in obtaining a job almost immediately, as a recreation therapist. She brings to the position an experience others cannot match, for she has very special insights into patient needs.

Shortly after L.'s discharge, I met a young man named G. who for three weeks refused to eat because he was convinced that staff were poisoning his food. During all that time he remained in his room. He seemed to me so dysfunctional, that I was certain that a state hospital would be his next destination, maybe his final destination. Well, nothing could have been further from the truth. One day, to my surprise, G. left his room and walked down the hall toward the recreation room. He walked very stiffly and slowly, because of his medication. When he came into the room I decided to offer him a simple activity, though I did not expect him to accept. I was quite wrong, however. He wasn't interested in chess, checkers, or dominoes, but he walked, almost as in a trance, over to our ping-pong table. Slowly, very slowly and awkwardly, his hand reached for the paddle, and the game began. This was more than a game of ping-pong. We were playing for keeps and the stakes were as high as they will ever be, in any game. I hit the ball high in the air, and slowly, so he could return it, at first; I was treating him with kid gloves, as a very casual opponent, when suddenly, without warning or expectation, the ball flew by me, and I lost the point. I returned to the table to begin the scenario once more; each time I returned and started a volley, each time the ball went back and forth, and then suddenly, out of nowhere the person on the other side of the table somehow managed to blast a shot by me.

As we played, we talked a little, slowly, getting acquainted. We only played about fifteen minutes the first day, twenty the second day, then thirty minutes. The quicker the ball went, the quicker and sharper was the conversation. We were playing the game of life, nothing less; no game was more intense, more serious, more thought out, or more fun. G. was recovering. The idea of a state hospital was now remote.

Prior to admission, G. had held his left arm over the stove, and left it there to burn, almost to the bone, because "the voices" told him to do it. Yet, with his good right arm, after three weeks of silence and morbidity, he played ping-pong with a stranger whom he had never met before. Ping-pong was a language he still remembered; with all his severe dysfunction and disturbance, G. could still be reached, but only if you spoke his language. G. later revealed to me that he had once been on the national ping-pong team of his country (Haiti). He went on to win every ping-pong tournament held on our unit.

To change sports, and challenge his eye-hand coordination, G. tried pool, now with his left hand recovering and less bandaged. Indeed, though many of our staff were adept at pool, none could defeat G. At his discharge, he went back to complete high school. He joined a track team and a wrestling team and started to volunteer in a nursing home. This is the man who the staff decided was on his way to the state hospital; the one who wouldn't speak, wouldn't eat, wouldn't "cooperate," as the staff put it. But he would *play*, if someone could believe in him enough to play with him. Playing this game means playing the game of life, and it is scary, because losing is serious business.

In January, 1982, I met a 25-year-old woman, P., recently admitted to our facility, and judged by staff as argumentative, hostile, hard to manage. She had many problems, but she responded to my invitation to come to our music therapy session. After a few sessions, it was P. who led the singing. To watch her sing and move about encouraging other patients was really an inspiration, so I asked her to leave her own ward and help me run music therapy on our second unit as well. This she did, gladly. Seeing that I appreciated her help, she soon started joining me in our daily calisthenics class as well. In fact she was so eager to help me that I had her help out with the typing in an outer office. When the time came for her discharge, I was able to help P. transfer to our Day Hospital. Since by this time she was typing 40 words per minute, she was able to obtain a job as well. I believe that P.'s successful role in helping with the recreation programs enabled her to believe in her ability to make it in the world outside the hospital.

Although many of our patients return to our psychiatric unit time after time, sometimes as often as five or six times a year, those I have described never returned. I believe that when patients can be successful at recreation it can give them hope for success in other areas of their life. Recreation is a natural intervention. It is part of peoples' lives outside the hospital; it is part of what "normal" people do. For that reason, I think, it is less threatening than some of the clinical approaches.

For recreation staff, sometimes this is a problem. They see the clinical approaches as more prestigious and can have a sense of inferiority at times—we are "only" recreation. The very thing that is our strength can be seen by others as a weakness, and sometimes we, too, accept this judgment. I believe this is a mistake. The patients I have described could only be reached by the naturalness, the simplicity, the unpretentiousness of recreation.